horses in translation

Essential Lessons in Horse Speak:
Learn to "Listen" and "Talk" in Their Language

sharon wilsie

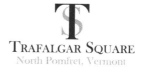

TRAFALGAR SQUARE
North Pomfret, Vermont

First published in 2018 by
Trafalgar Square Books
North Pomfret, Vermont 05053

Copyright © 2018 Sharon Wilsie

All rights reserved. No part of this book may be reproduced, by any means, without written permission of the publisher, except by a reviewer quoting brief excerpts for a review in a magazine, newspaper, or website.

Disclaimer of Liability

The author and publisher shall have neither liability nor responsibility to any person or entity with respect to any loss or damage caused or alleged to be caused directly or indirectly by the information contained in this book. While the book is as accurate as the author can make it, there may be errors, omissions, and inaccuracies.

Trafalgar Square Books encourages the use of approved safety helmets in all equestrian sports and activities.

Library of Congress Cataloging-in-Publication Data
Library of Congress Cataloging-in-Publication Data
Names: Wilsie, Sharon, author.
Title: Horses in translation : essential lessons in horse speak : learn to
   listen and talk in their language / Sharon Wilsie.
Description: North Pomfret, Vermont : Trafalgar Square Books, 2018. |
   Includes index.
Identifiers: LCCN 2017059447| ISBN 9781570768590 (paperback) | ISBN
   9781570769078 (ebook)
Subjects: LCSH: Horses--Behavior. | Human-animal relationships. |
   Human-animal communication.
Classification: LCC SF281 .W547 2018 | DDC 636.1--dc2
3LC record available at https://lccn.loc.gov/2017059447

Book design by Tim Holtz
Cover design by RM Didier
Typefaces: Cantoria, American Typewriter, Avenir, Josefin Sans, Quorum

Front cover and back cover main photos of Apache, loved by Mackenzie Menia, © Kristin Lee Photography; author photo by Francis Janik

Printed in the United States of America

10 9 8 7 6 5 4 3

This book is dedicated to the horses I have met
on this journey and who continue to educate, inspire,
and enlighten me as I endeavor to learn their language.

In loving memory of Zeke.

Contents

Acknowledgments

I would like to acknowledge my partner Laura for her tireless devotion to this work, and also my family and friends for all the help, love, and support they have provided. I also want to thank the wonderful and dedicated staff at Trafalgar Square Books. Furthermore, I want to say a big thank you to the horse-and-human partnerships that are the heroes and inspiration behind this book.

"How do you do? I'm looking forward to having this personal visit with you. Won't you sit down, and relax, while I deliver the master keys for unlocking the secrets for achieving your dreams?"
—Napoleon Hill, Author of *Think and Grow Rich*

Part One

read this first

Chapter 1

Introduction

Since my first book *Horse Speak: The Equine-Human Translation Guide* was published, I have had the opportunity to meet and work with hundreds of people and horses from all over the world. My fluency in "Horse Speak"—a practical system for "listening" and "talking" to horses in their language, instead of expecting them to comprehend ours—has deepened, but so has my understanding of what horses are usually the most confused about.

This book is dedicated to those horse lovers who are tirelessly trying to improve not only their relationship with their horses, but also with themselves. When you begin to have conversations with horses, they begin to converse with you—and most of what they are trying to tell people is that they wish their humans would feel the same sense of deep well-being that they as horses are capable of.

Time and time again I have witnessed horses at a clinic finding or returning to what I call "Zero"—the state of being present in the moment, being aware and calm—then turning around almost immediately and offering to share this newfound confidence with not only their owners, but every person in the arena. Be they Minis or Shires, breeding stallions, yearlings, or ancient school horses still depended on for their surefooted care, all cases have demonstrated horses whose first inclination is to offer a beautiful connection back to their humans as soon as they can.

Frequently, people have pulled me aside after a clinic to utter their amazement at the seeming simplicity of the "conversations" they are now having with their horses. "That's *it*? It seems so…easy…" are words I have heard hundreds of times.

Learning Horse Speak takes time in the same way that learning any new language takes time. A new language is not only about word equivalences. Becoming truly fluent in another language means you must also understand the nuances, subtle meanings, and even the *feel* of the word's implications.

Language represents each individual's point of view, expresses what is valued, and demonstrates emotional preferences. This is also true for Horse Speak.

I often equate Horse Speak to the skills required to drive a car: You must use all your body parts to drive a car. Your field of vision must be trained to scan the road itself, the areas on each side of the road, and any and all signs. You are expected to interpret dozens of even more subtle things. Yet, to seasoned drivers, all of this has become so commonplace that we can also talk to our passengers or tune in our radio without a second thought. Similarly, I have been guilty of carrying on a conversation with a horse at a clinic, only to be halted by the audience, who lost the gist of the dialogue. But it *can* become so familiar to you that, like me, you lose yourself in wonderful, interesting, often eye-opening discussions with your horse.

Who Are You?

If you are reading this book, then you are a "seeker." The horse that inspired you to take this path could be a scared-to-death rescue you just want to do right by or a soured, angry horse you hope to restore to sanity. Possibly it is your favorite riding horse—maybe he seems okay in general but leaves you with a nagging feeling that you are missing something. Perhaps you are just the type of person who always wants to "go deeper" and know more, or you are a professional who wants to have a better handle on the needs of your four-legged clients. You may have run the gauntlet of trainers, probably even learning valuable lessons along the way, yet still you remain dissatisfied—unfulfilled in some elusive way.

In working with hundreds of horse-human combinations, I can safely say that "what is missing" always revolves around one simple thing: *understanding*. Most people have a certain level of understanding when it comes to specific elements of horse care and horse training, and some people may be enjoying a certain amount of success with horses and with riding, but often "The Gap" still shows up…and then here you are, reading another book, seeking answers.

The Gap

What is "The Gap"? It is that nagging zone between *what we know* and *what we don't know* when it comes to horses.

Most people have some level of intuition, common sense, and just enough feel to "get the job done." I was one of these, with sufficient awareness and skill to get the job done for quite some time. I was doing good work, teaching Equine Assisted Learning and riding lessons at a college for students with learning disabilities. I was also the intercollegiate coach there for about four years. I had enough of the "right stuff" to carry a workload of private clients who varied from dressage and hunter-jumper riders to those who preferred Western pleasure to some who just wanted to trail ride bareback—even a few who drove. I worked with blind horses and horses that had suffered major head trauma, as well as starvation, abuse, and neglect cases. I taught volunteer trainings at local rescues and therapeutic riding centers, finding meaning in working with horses and riders who were often considered the toughest cases.

No matter what sort of horse-and-rider combination I found myself working with, at a certain point The Gap would show up.

The Gap is the chasm that eats up a person's confidence, leaving the horse misunderstood and stranded on the other side. The Gap is that odd feeling lurking in the back of an honest person's mind—the admission that you are not entirely certain what a particular horse is thinking. Perhaps you have success with 90 percent of the horses you work with and the The Gap is just that last 10 percent. Or maybe you are a new horse owner and The Gap skulks in your mind from sunup to sundown.

Even with all my success stories and my ability to make a living working with horses and their people, The Gap was eating away at me, too.

Partnership

I had horses I'd trained to not only walk to the mounting block on their own, but to lower their bodies and help "scoop" me onto their backs. Yet, I was still suffering from a nagging sensation that I could not be entirely sure that, given the choice, a horse would *ever* offer to do these sorts of things of his own accord.

The "buzz word" hitting the horse world at the time was "partnership." At first I was hooked by the idea of a partnership with my horse, like everyone else, because the word implies an orientation toward a connection that was *shared* and hosted a certain amount of camaraderie. After chewing on the word for a few years and seeing what passed for partnership in the industry, I started to have my doubts. After all, you can have partnership in a business, your personal life, or in sports and not actually *like* the other players. Partnership *implies* connection but does not necessarily deliver.

What, then, was I looking for? Whatever it was that *I* was seeking, I knew my students and clients were seeking it, too.

So...What Are We Looking For?

Ultimately, The Gap drove me like an unreachable itch to take time off to learn. At first, I honestly just sat around and stared, and struggled to get my preconceived notions to leave me alone.

I am an avid learner, which is why I love to teach. I had already absorbed a great deal of both classical and contemporary beliefs about horses: ideas about equine body language and how to train them. However, I had found that all too often, the available information about horses seemed to veer between too extremes: the idea that they are inherently lazy and bullies and must be made to work to another idea that they are so sentient we should not even be riding them.

I wanted to drink from a deeper well. The day the shift happened for me was the day I was reading in the pasture and my horse took the book I was reading (which was about horses) out of my hands and looked deeply into my eyes. In a flash of understanding, I got it. I had to ask horses, not humans, how to speak "horse."

Slowly, the light began to dawn: in my own small herd of horses of different ages, sexes, backgrounds, I would see a certain movement offered at a specific juncture, time and time again. Patterns began to emerge, and as I recorded those patterns, new ones would crop up that were even more nuanced. Eventually, I needed to have "bookends" to these "conversations" I was observing. In other words, I wanted to know: How do horses begin to speak with each other and how do they end? Furthermore, I needed to understand what horses valued—whatever each horse was seeking was what the conversation he or she was having was about...so what where they all seeking? Although many horse conversations seemed to revolve around their main concerns—safety, food, water, shelter, and pecking order—it soon became obvious to me that they had a very intricate body language that allowed them to convey quite a lot of meaning with a single ear twitch. My goal became to figure out what those movements were *exactly and specifically*.

Finally, I also needed to understand horses' patterns of hierarchy—not the simplistic "dominant" and "submissive" roles that have been handed out by behaviorists and horse trainers for years, but the actual minute-to-minute, play-by-play movements of a herd's life together.

What emerged was the reality that horses are always communicating, not just eating grass mindlessly. Every single movement is a comment of sorts. Yes, a horse swished at a fly…but *how* did he swish? Was it dramatic, emphatic, or rhythmical? Maybe he was just talking to himself about that fly, or maybe he was telling someone else nearby, "Hey, bad flies over here."

What it came down to was that horses can ask for company and they can ask for space. They can apologize after being grumpy. They can hold a line with an unruly youngster or gently guide the elderly. While human beings may be able to see when those interactions have happened, most of us have not come to realize *exactly and specifically* what movements happened when, why, and how to signal each portion of the continuous conversation that can be flowing between several horses at one time.

Becoming the Mother

In a herd, I found that "Mentors" can heal the lost souls or teach the young, but "Mothers" are the first and truest teachers, and all other roles spring off from the lessons a horse's dam taught him. If we emulate the Mother, we regain a horse's confidence, trust, and respect while also building rapport and encouraging bonding. The best Mentor horses are incredibly nurturing, calm, and steady. The best "Leaders" make sure all members of the herd are cared for and that they know that the Leader has their backs. The "Sentry" con-stantly assesses the environment. The "Bully" keeps everyone on his toes. The "Joker" lightens things up and the "Scaredy-Cat" keeps everyone alert. But the Mother was the first guide, and her communication style is the best one to copy if we want our horses to be both respectful and deeply bonded to us in a way that makes them feel completely at peace.

In this book, I challenge previously held beliefs about the word "leader-ship." For many the term has come to mean being the "boss." This image tends to place people in a certain mindset, which leads to a competitive, dominance-based relationship with their horses. What I have discovered is that to be a truly effective Leader with the horse is to consider oneself to be a teacher or coach. The horse's first teacher, first Leader, first coach, and first Mentor was his mother. The relationship between mother and foal instills a wide variety of values, from deep nurturing to strong healthy boundaries. Since what many of us want is to have a deep rapport with our horses—in an equation where both sides are balanced and satisfying—then picturing the qualities of the Mother can serve as a guide to help us become the best version of ourselves.

The bottom line for me came when my previously unhappy, hard-to-reach horse casually walked to the gate that led out to the trail through the woods on my land. Looking over his shoulder at me, he blinked his eyes, wiggled his lips, nodded his head, and blew out a big breath. I had nothing in my hands, so I simply took off my scarf, wrapped it around his neck, and opened the gate. He led me to the downed tree we often used if I was mounting bareback, and he blew out his nose, nodding his head as he squared up his feet. As I rose up to get on him, he leaned into my body to steady me. After I had settled on his back, he marched off at a nice pace, careful to give me room near the saplings that threatened my legs. We walked about halfway down the trail—20 minutes or so—then he paused, blew out, and looked back over his shoulder. I looked back that way, too, and he comfortably turned around and walked back to the pasture gate. All the while, I was breathing in deeply, listening to the tromp of his hooves, and marveling at this beautiful offer.

The answer I had found was, "Yes." Horses *will* offer, of their own accord, to carry us on their backs. All we need to learn to do is really listen.

How to Use This Book

This book is different from my first book, *Horse Speak: The Equine-Human Translation Guide*, which provided step-by-step instructions, explaining how to have what I call "conversations" with your horse, along with full-colored photographs to visually demonstrate both the horse's and the human's roles. This book is a collection of stories based on real events that are intended to help demonstrate how Horse Speak helps, *as well* as how it works. (Note: The names and some details have been altered to protect people's privacy, but the essence of each story remains.)

I find that storytelling is a wonderful way to really express the way Horse Speak works. Let me explain: Horses are highly ritualized—they follow patterns of actions and behavior—and once I started pulling those rituals together, I could observe the order in which a horse would use them to "ask questions" and "give answers." Horses can accomplish this in a matter of minutes, but humans need to have it all broken down into parts so we can learn the protocols related to their means of communicating with each other. The protocols or "rules" of Horse Speak are used and repeated whenever there is something to be negotiated between members of a herd. (I like to think of their language as a circular pattern rather than a linear one.) So in each story that lies ahead, I go through the protocols in detail as I uncover the source of a horse's distress, confusion, or frustration. The story provides a real scenario that makes it easy for each of us to relate and to apply the questions and answers to our own horses.

Before I share the stories, however, I have outlined my philosophy and seven key aspects of Horse Speak in chapters 2 and 3. Even if you have read my first book, I encourage you to peruse this section because I have shared new and evolving ideas about Horse Speak—things I have learned and pondered over the past year that may give you new insight or provide a breakthrough related to a concept you didn't quite "get" before.

Then, as you read the stories that follow, try to look for both the *science* and the *art* of the conversations I describe. The mechanics of movement (the science of body language) are designed to line a person up to be more clear and focused and calm in the presence of horses. The art of Horse Speak shows up as I dig down through the layers to help both the horses and the humans to find their "Zero." (Remember, this is the state of being present in the moment, being aware and calm. I talk more about what this means for horse and human on p. 37.) I highlight an "Aha Moment" in each story—that point where I, or another, finally understood what a horse was trying to communicate and how best to resolve the issue. In addition, each story ends with what I call the "Lick and Chew": key takeaways from the story that you can use in your day-to-day interactions with your horse, and which will result in exciting new levels of connection and communication.

To understand how horses really think and why they use the patterns they do, we first need to stretch ourselves outside of our own box of beliefs. Horse Speak is an honest attempt to authentically interact with horses in a manner similar to how they interact with each other, following the same protocols as they do. I acknowledge that I am not a horse. I am also not a dog, yet most people would agree that we can communicate quite a lot with one. Dogs have largely adapted to pay attention to our body language and verbal cues. All I am suggesting is that it is possible for *us* to adapt and pay attention to the horse's body language and *non*verbal cues.

It is my hope that the stories in this book convince you to stretch outside your box of beliefs.

Chapter 2

Horse Speak Philosophy

The beginning of learning Horse Speak starts when we allow ourselves to go beyond *looking* to truly *seeing*.

As human beings, we like to talk about stuff, name stuff, and we like to tell stories about stuff. However, horses do not objectify the way we do. We name everything, and knowing the names of things gives us a certain sense of control and power over the world. If we walk into a room, our brain names all the objects there—door, window, wall, rocking chair, book, cat, and so on— because when we "know what that is," we no longer fear it. Just think: If you were abducted by aliens and opened your eyes to find yourself on a spaceship, imagine how terrifying it would be to look around at a bunch of strange objects and not be able to identify them.

We use our reason to objectify and generalize the world and do not need a direct experience of things to understand them. Horses, however, are the opposite of this. They exist in a river of experience that they are constantly aware of—and commenting about. They are sensory machines. All their senses are firing at high levels to keep them constantly hyper-aware of their environment. So, if a horse expresses concern about his world right in the middle of a "conversation" we are having with him, all other thoughts must be put on hold while we address his concerns. Luckily, the more successful we are in retraining ourselves to do this, the more secure horses feel about the world. This brings nearly an end to spooking, and when a spook does happen, horses tend to regroup with us, rather than believing they need to escape from us.

> "I am a firm believer that without speculation, there is no good and original observation."
> —Charles Darwin, 1857

Learning to Observe

It is common practice to look at a horse and immediately analyze his features or parse what he can or can't do. We need to realize that fixating on a horse's features, for example, limits our ability to show up the way a horse needs us to—present, honest, and calm.

I have often told an owner not to talk about her horse right in front of him. If she wants to tell me a story about his behavior, I suggest we do it outside the barn. On countless occasions I have witnessed a horse begin pinning his ears, prancing around, and fidgeting as his human gets stirred up and fixated on the details of the horse's backstory. Horses are masters at observing proprioceptive shifts—the almost imperceptible changes in our bodies when we get emotional. We must attempt to observe *the horse's* micro-movements, too, but many people find it challenging to stop the internal dialogue and just *be present*, allowing themselves to see what is really there, in front of them, without editorializing. Learning to observe without a "little note-taker" in the back of your mind, comparing everything to everything else and asking, "Why?" all the time, takes practice. Taking notes and asking "Why?" in a broader context is fine, but the goal here is to try to suspend it while you are learning to observe.

> As soon as a child learns to talk, he also learns what "Don't touch that!" means. Horses still want to touch everything. When we don't allow some space for their exploration, or a way to tell them we think the objects are safe, they may grow more fearful.

Is This Anthropomorphism?

What I am attempting to do may seem to fly in the face of what some consider traditional core beliefs about horses.

Wikipedia defines *scientific method* as follows: "By reducing complex systems to smaller parts, scientific method is a body of techniques for investigating phenomena—acquiring new knowledge, or correcting and integrating previous knowledge with new criteria … using a method of inquiry to attain… empirical or measurable evidence." All I have attempted to do is take the complex system of horse body language and reduce it to smaller parts. The evidence shows up as the horses respond authentically to the human version of horse body language.

I am not a scientist, but I enjoy science and find its logic attractive. In fact, my mother was a veterinary technician when I was growing up, and I spent most of my free time hanging out with her at the family-run clinic, when I wasn't sick myself. Growing up handling animals in distress and surrounded by medical practices gave me a deep respect for science. Having spent much of my own childhood in oxygen tents and plugged into IVs, I instinctively knew to reach out to the sick animals with care and understanding. Through lessons and observation, I learned far more than just how to "pat the kitty"—I found out how to handle animals in distress and how to read the signs and signals that might indicate you are about to get bitten or scratched.

Of course, as much as I appreciate the wonders science has brought to us in terms of medicine, the fact is that in the name of science some horrible experiments were performed on animals for many years. This practice engendered the idea that animals are no more than groupings of behaviors and reactions to stimuli, and therefore, "beneath" humans. For a scientist to show compassion when involved in that sort of research was for him to be considered "un-objective," and likely tainting the results of the experiment by projecting his inner conflict, preferences, and emotions onto the object or animal in question.

> "If we feel ourselves emotionally affected by the behavior of an animal, it is a clear indication that we have intuitively discovered a similarity between its behavior and human behavior. We should not conceal this in our description."
> —Konrad Lorenz, Here am I—Where Are You? (Collins, 1991)

Conversely, we have a compulsion to truly anthropomorphize animals all over the place: we give them human characteristics, thoughts, and behaviors in children's books, television commercials, and movies, on social media—you name it. Many argue humans need to feel connected to nature, and in the void created by urban living and technology-driven lifestyles, we have found a way to allow our feelings space by creating fantasy images of animals.

We base most of our decisions on feelings, and whether we like it or not, we can get offended or frustrated with horses simply because we have assigned them anthropomorphic qualities: "He knows what he should do, he's just being stubborn." "Don't let him get away with it, he's trying to fool you." "Horses are inherently lazy—you must get after them." "He's not respecting you."

And: "He's my big baby!" "He takes such good care of me." "He's such a ham." And so on and so forth.

These are all common misinterpretations of behavior seen in the horse world, and they unfortunately drive a great deal of what we do with our horses.

The fact is, we anthropomorphize because both humans and horses are mammals and we both have feelings: attachments, conflicts, and the desire to feel safe, as a few examples. But when we assign human emotions to a horse's reactions, that is often where the source of conflict comes in (and The Gap shows up). The problem is *not* whether an animal's feelings are valid in a laboratory—none of us lives in a laboratory! The problem is reading and interpreting animal body language for what it is as accurately as we can without dumping our preconceived notions all over it.

Horses not only have feelings, they are feeling-based creatures. The way they feel is one of the things that draws us to them. Horses have horse emotions, and humans have human ones, but together we can share the best of ourselves, when we learn how. What Horse Speak offers is a way to clarify both our observations and our ability to interpret them.

> "Fear of the dangers of anthropomorphism has caused ethologists to neglect many interesting phenomena, and it has become apparent that they could afford a little disciplined indulgence."
> —Robert Hinde, *Ethology* (Oxford University Press, 1982)

Where Rapport Comes From

Most of us are not involved in scientific equine research, nor are we in a cavalry regiment. In cavalry training, horses and riders went through boot camp together. They also lived together, which nurtured the intense bonds that comrades form under such circumstances. I have seen some touching black-and-white photos from the turn of the century in which cavalry soldiers and their horses appear to be demonstrating what I would call a very deep rapport with each other.

However, in our modern world, the majority of us show up to ride our horses a few times a week, at most. Even if riding lessons are treated like military schooling, it still does not have the same effect it would if the horse and rider were living and working together and relying on each other in the way they would if they were in boot camp—laboring together, eating, sleeping, cleaning up together, and enjoying leisure time, too...*together*. Consider the police dog, who must live with his handler full time to attain the depth of relationship necessary for the dog's continued and sustained effort in his work. The desire for an obedient, "push-button" response from horses (and ourselves) when handling or riding them, when the relationship has not had the benefit of being cultivated and nurtured, is sure to be disappointed.

In lieu of the time and energy it would take to actively live, day in and day out, in the sort of scenario likely to create that depth of relationship we crave, we have come to rely upon methods or systems that are still *based* on obedience but *aim* for communication. There are *many* "modern" horsemanship techniques out there that promise a safe, willing horse if you follow their rules just right. However, safe and willing is not truly attainable if the horse has not given his heart over to you. The *outside* of a horse can certainly be drilled into compliance, but the inside of a horse is a whole other thing…

The challenge with horses, as I have come to understand it, is that we want two opposing values to be reached: we want obedience, but we also want love. *Obey me* and *love me* are two entirely different expectations.

I have experienced horses who have incredible loyalty and would work for me all day long, but my goal is to also reach the "inner self" of those horses and create a situation in which their skin and heart is in the game *with* me… not in obedience *to* me. This may sound like a picky word choice, but sometimes tiny shifts in awareness create a waterfall of change.

> "It's categorically wrong to say that animals don't have thoughts and emotions, just like it's wrong to say they are completely the same as us."
> —Carl Safina, *Beyond Words: What Animals Think and Feel* (Picador, 2016)

While on the Subject of Words...

I am using some catch phrases in this body of work that will certainly sound like anthropomorphizing, and there is a reason for that. I am working with the communication system of horses and there are quite a few groupings of signals within that. It is necessary to assign labels both in order to learn the system and to gain a feeling of what its intricacies in fact mean.

For instance, I use the term "Aw-Shucks" to refer to the horse lowering his head to touch his muzzle to the ground when he is not eating. This signal is a comment about pressure or tension or intensity. If the horse lowers his head while approaching you, he is lowering the pressure to not offend you, in the same way he would when approaching another horse. If you are approaching him, and he lowers his head and tucks it to the side, he may be asking you to slow down or decrease your energy. If he lowers his head and sniffs your boot, he may be commenting on how close you are standing to him—he may feel crowded and is asking your feet to please move back and away. There are many more examples and many nuances, so I simply call this action "Aw-Shucks" to remind the human thinking of that phrase to lower his or her intensity. I am not suggesting the horse is actually saying or thinking, "Aw-Shucks." Honestly, I could have just called it "Lower the Intensity," but that sounds boring.

> My experience with Horse Speak has been a "clearing of the mist"—a sort of awakening, if you will. Once a person catches on to the basic system, the results that the horses offer are consistently positive and consistently lasting.

Each term I use in Horse Speak is a catch phrase intended to remind us of not only the grouping of signals, but also the right feeling to apply to that grouping. To take a visual language (how horses communicate) and turn it into verbal language (phrases we understand) so that we can approximate the mechanical and energetic effect of a signal is not easy. In fact, if you want to call the signals something else, be my guest!

The bottom line here is that my aim is not to only teach methods that resonate with and are understood by a crowd of behaviorists at a university; I want to help *everyone*.

The Nature of Language

So what is *language* anyway?

According to Wikibooks contributors to the text *Introduction to Linguistics*, "Language is a system for communicating. Written languages use symbols (that is, characters) to build words. The entire set of words is the language's vocabulary. The ways in which the words can be meaningfully combined is defined by the language's syntax and grammar. The actual meaning of words and combinations of words is defined by the language's semantics."

When it comes to *animal* versus *human* communication, contributors go on to say: "Systems of communication are not unique to human beings. Other animal species communicate in a variety of ways. One way is by sound… Another means of animal communication is by odor… A third means of communication is body movement, for example used by honeybees to convey the location of food sources.

"Communication can be defined to include both signals and symbols. Signals are sounds or gestures that have a natural or self-evident meaning [example of someone crying (=emotion), laughing (=emotion), animal cries (=indicating fear, food, or hunt)…. Animal communication tends to consist primarily of signals."

You have already heard me use the term "signal" in my previous discussion of how horses communicate. I suggest that Horse Speak is in fact a form of language, not a new form of behaviorism.

Behaviorism, as it applies to training animals, seeks only to gauge observable reactions or responses. In *strict* behavioral theory, you cannot calculate the inner workings of the mind or emotions, only measurable (that is, viable) aspects of whatever an animal is *doing*. Behavior you want versus behavior you don't want is the basis of any training methodology. With enough coercion, consequence, or reward, animals can be coaxed into memorizing the patterns of behavior that we seek.

For example, B.F. Skinner was a behaviorist who worked with *operant conditioning*, in which subjects were offered levels of rewards, from simple to high-value, with clear indicators and markers to allow the subjects to know when they had completed the task. He was interested in reward-based conditioning because the *pleasure response* can overrule most inclinations to resist. There was a fascination with moveable parts of machinery at the time, and the workings of life were linked to "cogs in a wheel." Behavior was supposedly just groups of reactions and responses to stimulus—no more, no less.

If this model were strictly true, then all horses could be trained using the exact same methods, and we would end up with the exact same results—cogs in a wheel—and we all know that is just not the case.

Decoding vs. Encoding

Horse Speak offers something different.

Body language makes up something like 80 percent of all communication. There are whole sciences now dedicated to decoding human facial expressions, postures, and gestures, and frame-by-frame photography shows micro-movements of the face that happen too fast to see with the naked eye but that our brains interpret anyway.

There are two main parts to the science of body language:

1. *Decoding* means the ability to process and understand the nonverbal cues being sent to you.

2. *Encoding* is *your* message: how you express yourself nonverbally to others (with the hope that they can decode you!)

The first part of learning Horse Speak revolves around *decoding*, and the second part involves your ability to *encode*. The third stage is the synthesis of decoding and encoding: when they come together, then the conversation flows. Some of you will pick it up in a day; others may need more time. However, I taught this to my Equine-Assisted Learning groups for many years, and without fail, after one semester, everyone walked away with a good working knowledge of it!

Rude

The words we use to describe what horses are doing are hardwired to also make us feel a certain way. Some have studied the use of words in an attempt to understand how they impact how we feel within ourselves and how we relate to the outside world. For instance, the word "money" elicits a certain feeling: For some it causes instant tension or a "clamping" sensation, possibly linked to feelings of anger or frustration or fear. For others, it causes an "open-ing" sensation and feelings of pleasure. Because of this, many financial advisors try to use other words like "funds" when they talk to clients; they wish to avoid the word that might trigger a negative reaction.

It is essential when analyzing your horse's actions that you pay attention to the words you use to describe them. Far too often, for instance, we assume a horse is "rude." This usually happens when he is doing something that we don't like. But if we slow down and just take the facts as they are, try to *really* see it from the horse's point of view, we may discover the word doesn't really fit the situation. In addition, using such words to describe actions we don't like or calling our horses derogatory terms like "jerk," "pig-headed," "beast," or "witch" (for example) sets up an emotional reaction inside us. Feelings are not facts, and facts are not feelings. The fact might be the horse spooked sideways when you tried to saddle him. Your feeling about that fact might be that it felt "dangerous," or "disobedient," or maybe "rude." You may even apply such words to your own actions ("I'm an idiot." "I'm stupid"). These feelings arise in reaction to the fact—they are *reactionary feelings*, but not the real ones. The real feelings that matter usually lie one layer deeper: You get scared, then you get angry, then you assign meaning to the encounter (the horse was bad, or you were bad). From there, you may slip into a *core belief*—an assumption you make about yourself, others, or the world that you mistake for fact (for instance, your horse doesn't love you or you aren't a good rider).

There is a saying that the horse is a reflection of ourselves; I would suggest that *the way we paint the image of the horse* is the reflection of ourselves. If all the horse does is become reactive and we label him as "rude," that says more about us than it does about him. Remember, horses are prey animals, and Mother Nature put those reactions in there for a reason.

If you can learn even a few basics of Horse Speak and hold onto a couple of simple points of awareness in relation to what horses value intrinsically, you can begin to lay these kinds of "go-to" assumptions to rest and enter into a conversation with your horse that is much more productive.

Science and Art

As I mentioned in chapter 1, Horse Speak is both a science and an art. There is a *science* to the mechanics of moving your body in specific ways to communicate. The *art* of Horse Speak develops when a person becomes fluent enough to respond to nuance.

For horses to believe our body language, we must match our insides with our outsides. Trying to hide an emotion—like fear, for example—will never work, because horses are uniquely clued in to the inner state of a predator species (that would be us). You cannot lie to a horse. It is, therefore, more useful to simply acknowledge and label the emotion you might be experiencing than to try to hide it or ignore it. Your horse does not care if you are feeling a particular emotion—he only cares that you are honest. Many of my students have found that by arriving at the barn and immediately telling the horses all about their daily stress, they feel better—and achieving congruency inside and out instantly calls the horses to them. When we line up our inside and outside, we find that state of Zero I mentioned back on page 11.

The "Leader" of the herd is the horse with the calmest nerves, the most attuned senses, and the sharpest mind. Horses do not thrive on stress; in fact, it wears them down. For a herd to be healthy, its members need to stay in that state of mind I call Zero. Because, as we've discussed, people have so many attachments to labels, words, and meanings, telling someone to "stay calm" may have the opposite effect. I use the word Zero to simply mean being in a state of inner calm; that is the kind of leadership your horse is looking for.

> The urge to control horses makes perfect sense; they are huge, emotional creatures capable of enormously athletic antics. Horses can be downright scary, and to deny this or try to act tough about it is to set yourself up for incongruent actions toward your horse: your insides and your outsides won't match. And your horse will know this.

Leadership

I am going out on a limb here and say that "training" and "leadership" may not always be the same thing when it comes to horses. Cultivating the behaviors you want by punishing or minimizing the unwanted behavior is a standard practice. With many trainers, there is also an emphasis on "making the right thing easy" or somehow rewarding the behaviors you want to see.

Leadership is not the same thing as dominance. No animal claims total dominion over another animal as a rule of thumb, except for humans. Within a herd, pack, or flock members all form links in a chain, and the strength of the community is the most important part of the whole. The most important element is *not*, as some believe, the "alpha role"—whatever that is. The man who coined the phrase "Alpha Wolf," David Mech, later recanted that idea. As his studies of wolves progressed, he came to understand that the behavior and roles in a pack were more nuanced and subtle.

In the wild, the strongest male is usually the one who earns breeding rights, which ensures good genes for the babies. Other than mating season, however, large males are not necessarily the leaders. Most often packs, herds, and other large groups have strong female leadership, or are entirely made up of females, as you find in elephant herds. The group focus is on mutual safety, camaraderie, and community. The daily life of most animal groups is concerned with getting enough food, shelter, water, and watching out for each other. Wild animals do not want to waste precious energy bickering, and social groups have a wide variety of systems to ensure the peace and quiet that supports the health and vitality of the group, and avoids attracting predators.

In chapter 1 I mentioned how Horse Speak teaches us to "become the Mother." Here's why: Leadership can be best witnessed by watching a mare and her foal. "Mom" is protective, nurturing, tolerant, yet also teaches her little one boundaries, rules, and—most importantly—how to communicate.

Our domestic horses live in box stalls, and in fields or paddocks that are surrounded by fences. There is a limited amount of experience young horses get out in the wide world. That is where we come in. If a horse has never been on a trail ride, his first one may be completely overwhelming. Mom never got to teach him how to handle the woods, or the rocks, or the fallen logs.

Horses map their surroundings in their heads; it is one of their survival skills. If Mom gets turned out in a new pasture with her baby, she scans the horizon, sniffs the fence-line, and tours the area to see what is what. If she tenses up for any reason during this exploration, her baby is supposed to freeze and wait for her to say, "All's clear!" or "RUN!"

The leadership role that is the easiest for humans to pick up and emulate is that of the mother. Note that this is *not* to be confused with treating your horse like a baby; in fact, "babyish" horses (like the 18-year-old Thoroughbred that acts like a yearling) will begin to "grow up" if you become "Mom." Taking on the leadership role that Mom left behind means you begin to finish fulfilling the horse's need to follow the most important being in his life. You will be able to influence boundaries, bonding, and decision-making. You will be able to use the same kind of leadership his mother did to help him make new maps of the world, learn better, and feel calmer and more centered (that all-important Zero).

With the wide variety of activities we usually expect our horses to participate in, offering the role of leadership that encapsulates clear, calm, assertiveness is a good idea.

"Xs" and "Os"

By adopting an "O" posture—rounded shoulders and arms, hands lightly touching, head and neck relaxed, and softened jaw and lips (tight lips makes it look like you might bite!)—your brain and nervous system get the signal, "All's clear, you're safe." This posture urges your inner state in the direction of Zero, causing you to breathe deeply. It is universally recognized as welcoming, beckoning, and softening.

The opposite of this is the "X" posture: high, tense shoulders, tight lips, hard eyes, breath held, tense legs. All of this signals the brain to be on alert and hyper-vigilant—away from a state of Zero. This posture sends adrenaline throughout our bodies and prepares us to fight, flee, or freeze.

In today's world, we tend to get stuck in one posture or the other: either in too much "X" or too much "O" (which is more like a slump). Depression, anxiety, childhood issues, stress, all lodge in our bodies. If too much time passes, we can reach the third stress response and freeze into either an "X" or "O," depending on our disposition.

However, if we begin to pay attention to our "Xs" and "Os," our Zero starts to show up more regularly.

The Horse's Zero

Many horses have lost their Zero due to long-term stress. Horses cannot find Zero for themselves once they've reached this point, but when we make the state of Zero our goal for ourselves in every situation, the horses find their way back, too.

Since they cannot usually either fight or flee from people, sometimes the domestic horse's response is to freeze in depression, confusion, or anxiety. He might also act out: Stomping, nipping, fidgeting, head-tossing, or rubbing on you are *always* indicative of a horse losing his Zero. A healthy, well-balanced horse does not need to "de-stress himself" by acting out.

Rather than starting by addressing each little issue with a horse (crowding, pawing, pacing the stall), I aim straight for returning him to Zero. I find problem behaviors often literally melt away as inner calm is returned to the horse. A calm horse is one who can pay attention, learn, and perform as a partner. He will offer to be *with* us in exchange for feeling this good in our presence.

To illustrate this, think about being a kid in school and getting called up to the front of the class to answer a question. The stress of being put on the spot might cause you to freeze; maybe you can't even remember the question. Standing there, sweating, panicking, and feeling worse by the moment is not a good association with the lesson. Now imagine the teacher starts yelling at you or belittling you for not knowing the answer!

"Trauma is not what happens to us, but what we hold inside in the absence of an empathetic witness."
—Peter A. Levine, Psychologist and Author

Most of us, however, had at least one teacher in school who was calm and understanding. That teacher might be fondly remembered, her image basked in a warm glow in your mind as you feel gratitude for the time you spent with her. Her own inner state of calm engendered the same in you, and this made it possible for you to not only learn more, but also eager to please and capable of performing better in the classroom.

When a horse is calm, he is happy. A happy horse uses his "O" posture to show this. If you help your horse feel happy, he will seek to please you and will offer so much in return.

Slow Way, Way Down

Horses are not machines, motorcycles, or computers. We tend to want a timely response, especially when we are riding at higher levels, but we need to remember that horses think *slowly* but react quickly. This often means we are getting reactive answers, not thoughtful ones. Over time, when a horse really *comprehends* a cue with everything in his being and is not afraid to execute that maneuver, he can practice doing it with speed. We have been taught that a horse must be "forward" first to have the essential impulsion, rhythm, and balance needed to perform; however, the horse is then only learning by rote, which does not allow him to contemplate the essence of the lesson. The risk of a horse in this situation being triggered into hyper-vigilance and survival mode is very close to the surface.

Slow way, way down to renegotiate everything you are trying to do or say to your horse. If you ask for something, wait for the thoughtful response, instead of pushing for the reactive one. Learn to *pause*.

> Horse Speak can be used as a diagnostic tool to uncover the real source of stress in a horse's life. When the horse feels better, he acts better, and he retains better health.

I also often suggest a person stay outside the stall, pen, or paddock, aiming her pointer finger toward the horse for a long time, and watch what happens. Just observe *without a purpose*. You will start to connect the dots for yourself when you witness the horse move in some way in a minute or two.

When you are done sending a message, be very careful to slowly remove the cue. If you have a confused, pushy, or fearful horse who reacts too quickly, then you need to use all your body movements as though you're swimming: slowly, rhythmically, and with a clear beginning and end.

Remember the saying, "Hurry slowly." The more you allow a conversation with a horse to unfold, in its own time, the more likely you will not have gaps and misunderstandings in your work together.

Horses Value Space

Remember this: *Balanced Boundaries Make Better Bonding*. Horses need their issues with personal space cleared up first; then they can practice getting close. Most horses are confused about how close is too close, or when we really want closeness and when we don't, so if your foundation is "personal space first," there is always a safe spot to retreat to for both of you.

Horses value space. Let me say that again: *Horses value space* more than food, water, shelter, comfort, and touch. If a horse does not have space to move, he cannot escape, and Mother Nature designed him to be a master of fleeing. When horses feel crowded by us, if we invade their "personal bubble" all the time, if we never let up on the pressure, they have no space.

When a horse steps away from you, turns his head away from you, or otherwise moves over for you, he is giving you room. Horses use space like money: when they really like you, they give you the thing they most covet—*space to be*. Horse Speak begins any conversation with carefully approaching a horse's "bubble of personal space." We don't even begin to say hello until we are welcomed to approach. When I tell a horse I care more about personal space than about touching him, I seem like a safer being to hang around with. Then, clearing up the confusion surrounding anything that

Do not just throw your arms back down into what you may assume is a neutral stance; this often looks like an "O" to a horse, and he may perceive it as an invitation to come into your space. When a horse tends to be so overreactive it is hard to accomplish even the small things, keep your body in a constant "X" that is not threatening but that tells him you want boundaries at all times. A horse will feel safer, faster when he knows the rules are not going to switch from boundaries to bonding and back to boundaries again without any understanding as to why that is.

bothers that horse is already set on a platform of deep mutual respect. I never need to force respect through heavy-handed tactics. Respect and connection happen simultaneously *because I value what the horse values*: safety in the world and clear personal boundaries. Horses give me respect because I am respectful of them.

How Does Horse Speak Influence Training?

I consider "training" whatever it is that you enjoy about horsemanship. Whether you like driving or trail riding or jumping or dressage, training is the "work" you ask your horse to perform with you.

Most of us work with other people, and we know there is a time to be busy and focused on the job, and there are also moments to "hang out at the water cooler" and talk. In addition, we know that when there is a work-related question, we of course must communicate with others to ask it as well as be prepared to receive and understand their answer. With Horse Speak, you should begin to be able to not only "hang out at the water cooler" and talk to your horse, but also decode what work-related questions your horse may have for you, then effectively communicate your answers back to him.

Although Horse Speak may cause you to re-evaluate what you are doing with your horse or how you are doing it, it doesn't necessarily need to be considered an alternative to the kind of training you prefer or enjoy. This education can supplement your riding, driving, or groundwork, allowing you to gain clarity and insight into how to help your horse develop the potential you feel he really has. Horse Speak will also help you become the person your horse needs you to be.

I have successfully applied Horse Speak in conjunction with a wide variety of training modalities. Frequently, riders gain a completely new perspective when it comes to their work with their horses. One man sat through an entire seminar, looking skeptical with his arms crossed, only to have such an eye-opening experience riding his horse using "Xs" and "Os" that he immediately wanted lessons. With Horse Speak, his horse found it easy to understand and perform the exercises that previously had caused the two the most trouble.

When a horse senses that you are *really trying* to understand him, he is frequently so grateful that he seeks connection with you in new and surprising ways.

Know Thyself

Horse Speak can help you and your horse reach the potential that you each have within you to become the best versions of yourselves. However, Horse Speak *cannot* magically turn your horse into a different horse.

If you want a German Shepard, don't buy a Poodle. Horses are who and what they are. As you grow together with your horse, you may need to re-assess what motivates you to be a horse person. We all have dreams in the backs of our minds, but we are still living in the here and now. Some dreams can come true, and some dreams are just the flashing light, pointing you in a direction you needed to go. But they are not the goal itself.

Of all the dreams I have ever heard people talking about, eventually most people realize that all they really want is to feel at home inside themselves and with their horses. Big goals are fun, and dreams that come true can be fun, too. But horses don't know about the picture in the back of your mind that they are supposed to live up to. By double-checking your agenda, you clear the path to be able to take a long walk with your horse with as much gusto as winning the grand prize. Maybe taking the long walk *is* your grand prize.

Misconceptions

When a person begins to use Horse Speak, a few misconceptions tend to emerge. We have all been acculturated to believe quite a few things about horse behavior that don't quite hit the mark. In golf, a tiny shift in your stance or your swing either sends the ball into the hole, or far away from it. The same holds true with horses.

Beliefs are a funny thing—we can hold on to an idea on the inside despite it not actually matching what is truly happening on the outside. Let me explain: Often people ask me questions like, "If I keep teaching this to my horse, will he learn it?" or "How long do you have to practice Horse Speak before they get it?" But Horse Speak is an attempt to use *their* body language cues, with the feel, timing, and "close-enough" gestures to calibrate a conversation with *them*. In other words, horses already use Horse Speak—they already desire to live at Zero and already want to have simple, clear boundaries that create simple, clear bonding.

The bottom line is that you are not teaching Horse Speak to your horse, you are learning it for yourself.

Forcing Relationship and Connection

You cannot force a relationship. You cannot *make* someone like you or love you or do what you want—aside from paying somebody a lot of money or owning a slave.

Forcing a horse to give us what we want does not make a relationship happen. We can force horses to give us a performance or work for us, but that is not a partnership. Forcing a horse over a jump he fears with a whip, then caressing his face or giving him an apple is incongruent. It is like saying, "I command you to obey me; now I command you to love me for it."

I am *not* saying horses do not take pride in or enjoy their work; they certainly may when it is presented the right way. However, if we approach a horse with the mixed message of, on the one hand, needing to feel love, connection, partnership, or affection, and on the other hand, needing the horse to boost our own ego or image with the perfect performance at a show or the best time in a race, then on neither hand have *we shown up for the horse*.

I want everyone to feel what it is like to have your horse line himself up at the mounting block with eagerness. I have asked horses to work for me in Equine-Assisted Learning classes, as riding school horses, as safe trail horses, as therapy horses, and as show horses. I have helped horses learn to enjoy their owners and whatever kind of "work" their owners are into. In almost every situation, I've seen horses come to a proud connection with that work once they see their people as the source of safety, connection, and loyalty. And if they could not connect to that work, then we found them another job that suited them better.

You can develop a horse's pride in his work with small, clear, achievable goals that you celebrate together with him. Take the two extra minutes to ask the horse when he is ready to leave his stall. Slow down your frantic pace. Stay honest about the horse in front of you and the dream you hold in your head and are trying to live up to.

Too often, I have witnessed a clinician forcing a horse to run around and sweat, but because the clinician succeeds in getting the horse to run onto a trailer he's afraid of or over a bigger jump, the audience is so overwhelmed by the showmanship that they forget to ask themselves, "Is this really okay?" A clinician might talk a good talk, but forcing horses, in whatever form it takes, is not pretty.

Frequently, people ask me, "How am I supposed to get anything done if I don't *make* it happen? It's not like the horse is going to saddle himself."

Think of a friend calling you mid-day to invite you to go out to lunch at a new bistro. You are busy doing other things and not sure you are ready to leave. Your friend knows you, and knows that you aren't partial to bistros, so she offers to pay for your lunch to help convince you to come. So you go and have a nice lunch, and in the end are glad you went—you were busy and not really into the idea but you put aside your projects and your reticence in order to connect with your friend and are glad for it. In fact, you may have even liked this bistro a little.

Now let's think of the same scenario, but your friend *insists* that you are going to lunch with her by showing up at your house and forcing you to put your shoes on. She belittles you, says you're no fun, and drags you to the car. Then she suggests you split the bill and proceeds to order more food than you do. You now know you *truly* hate bistros and spend the whole time wishing you were at home finishing your projects.

We all need a little prompting, sometimes. The choice is in how you do it.

Running to Think

There is unfortunately a wide-spread belief throughout today's horsemanship world that states plainly that horses must "move their feet" in order to think.

That golf metaphor applies here once again: a millimeter off your golf swing sends your ball right into the sand trap. What *is* true is that horses move their entire body to communicate. I am a person who often needs to talk out loud to process my inner thoughts; other people are quiet and keep a lot inside. The same holds true for horses: the body is their communication tool, they must use the body to talk, and some horses are just more talkative than others.

However, this is where the reality of horse body language and the misconceptions I've outlined on previous pages bang heads. When a horse is blinking, he is thinking. We all know the eyes show the "soul of the horse." It is also true that the eyes show the thinking processes of the horse. Wide, staring eyes show he is too stressed to think—hyper-vigilance has kicked in. "Tented" eyes show worry, fear, or concern. Cold, hard eyes show distance or even disassociation. Hard eyes with flat back ears often mean the horse is under the control of the fight-or-flight reflex—when you get this look from a horse, you may have done nothing wrong, but he is not present with you anymore.

Ears demonstrate the small fluctuations in the horse's thoughts and feelings. In fact, for many horses, backward-pointing ears are a sign of deep concentration, not necessarily aggression. When you see a horse really sorting things out, or paying attention to the rest of the herd or the world, you will often see backward-pointing ears. Our human body language equivalent is frowning as we concentrate while taking a test. If the ears are pointed backward, the head rises, and the lips get tight, then the horse may be right on the edge of what he can understand or handle. He is trying to concentrate but starting to lose it. He might be frustrated. Ears laid *flat* back are angry or extremely defensive. Sideways (airplane) ears are soft and relaxed, and inward-pointed ears are somewhere between concentrating and relaxed. Perky ears are just that: perky. Combined with a high head, they can mean a high-energy eagerness ("Can't wait!") or concern ("Ye gads!"). Perky ears and a low head are eager, but careful, or even beckoning with both desire and softness.

One of the most misunderstood gestures is when a horse turns his head quietly to the side. This is the horse's sign of respect. Remember, he uses space like a commodity. Giving you space is showing you respect, not leaving the area. When a horse carefully touches your boot, or your shoulder, he is asking you to stop crowding him. He prefers you to stand in the "buddy up" zone at his shoulder once you are all done sorting out who's who with his head space.

Horses *do* use their feet as part of their communication system, but the truth is that frequently this is narrowed down to a single step at a time. One step toward a horse or one step away carries significance! Asking a horse to move a single foot, pausing, then asking for one more single step will create the quiet, thoughtful, focused awareness that we are really after because this is what horses do with each other. All day, every day, they are moving and communicating. That grazing, munching, and stepping that we all take for granted is part of an overture of conversation that is flowing right along between them. If a horse can focus with us the way he focuses with his herd mates, the work we want to do with him suddenly becomes much simpler to achieve.

The bottom line is, when horses are thinking, they *slow down*, they don't speed up. If horses react, it is like lightning, but when they sort something out, they need time. Therefore, I teach people to leave a single cue in the air for a full minute sometimes. When you give horses a full minute to sort it all out, they can reply in a calm, focused manner, and that is when it all starts to feel good. Once they clearly comprehend your message, they will reply more quickly next time.

Speeding a horse up does wear off an amount of adrenaline so that the horse gets tired. Or it runs off his initial reaction, and so the horse starts looking for a way out. Occasionally, moving forward at a trot or canter with three quick changes of direction is therapeutic in a moment of stress or confusion. This is like when a person needs to burst out and talk for a few minutes about something on her mind. Her friends don't mind the first time, but they want to help her work through it; they don't want to hear about the same issue over and over again.

If you *must* round pen or longe or liberty run your horse to get a conversation started or to arrive at the point at which you can work, then you and your horse are spinning the same story over and over again. He has no chance to find the source of his stress and confusion, and neither do you. We shouldn't need to fix our horses every day. We need to find our Zero and their Zero, and then they will start to sort *themselves* out.

Making the Wrong Thing Hard

There is another popular thought in the horse world today that has gotten a little confused. This idea is to make the wrong thing hard for a horse and make the right thing easy. This is supposed to encourage a horse to choose the correct path.

While this principle is not inherently bad, the actions one takes to create it can be. Humans are instinctively inclined to want control, so by making the wrong thing hard, we emphasize *hard*. How is something a true "choice" when the alternative is terrible?

I once watched a trainer using this idea to teach a horse to do a spin, turning on the haunches very quickly. He rode in tighter and tighter canter circles until the only option left for the horse was to use his front end exclusively. The idea that the horse was somehow making any sort of choice about performing the right way for his trainer would be incorrect. There are no "choices" when the activity is forced. I've watched the same principle at work in a jump school: if the horse hit a rail or missed the distance, he was cantered in repeated circles around the obstacle, many times without letting up, then aimed at the jump again. When the horse made it clear, he got to rest. And in a liberty work demonstration, a trainer swished a rope and clucked loudly, cantering her horses over jumps repeatedly until finally, the pressure came off and the horses were allowed to come to the trainer, rest, and then follow her around. The "choice" was go out there and work hard and sweat, or stay in here with me where you get to be quiet.

We have a culture of starting off the "partnership" with a horse by making him sweat. This basically teaches the horse that when I show up, *you, horse, better get ready to freak out, because only after freaking out will I allow you to stand quietly with me.* This whole philosophy is based on the idea that if you put two horses together who don't know each other, one will chase the other until the other submits. It is true that occasionally there is quite a lot of scuffle between two horses, but the reasons and the degrees of nuance involved are usually quite lost to the human onlooker. All we see is one horse run and sweat hard and the other seem to "win." I argue that there are plenty of times you turn a new horse out with others, there is a brief greeting, and all involved settle down together just fine, without any running at all. The philosophy based on moving a horse's feet to achieve dominance falls apart, then.

I suggest changing the common phrase to: "Make the right thing *so* easy that the wrong thing feels harder." Then we come closer to what this idea is really based on. When we witness a gifted horseperson, most of us say something like, "He makes it look so easy." *That* is the point. It *is* easy, if *easy is your focus*. Not "hard."

What you focus on is what you create.

Look at the Pony

Too often, we see a performance of one sort or another, and we are looking at the power, beauty, or level of training of a horse. We are "looking at the pony," feeling the "wow" factor, but perhaps not tuned in to what is underneath. Taking the time to understand and use Horse Speak means you will start to see through any Wizard-of-Oz cleverness: Who is really behind the curtain? Is there a feeling of joy or stress? What does a happy horse really *look* like?

A happy horse uses his "O" posture to show contentment. Excitement does not inherently mean happiness. Excitement can appear fun, but one can be excited and scared, as well. Happiness for a naturally intense animal like a horse means that his nervous system is not all fired; it means he is deeply relaxed.

When I play rousing liberty games with my horse Dakota, she may enjoy rearing or trotting a half-pass or rolling a big ball. Her face may look almost fierce, with backward-facing, concentrating ears, and an arched, high poll. However, as soon as the intensity is over, it is over: if I hold my palm toward her forehead and nod my head downward, blowing out a deep breath, she lowers her head, and blows out, too. We never lost Zero just because we became exuberant. Her happy place is to stand very still, breathing deeply with me, and maybe licking my palm.

When a horse has his Zero, then any other kind of performance you seek to enjoy with him is truly a shared experience because both horse and human are deeply connected on the *inside*, not just doing something together on the outside. This is where it all begins.

Chapter 3

7 Keys to Horse Speak

In the last chapter, I described many of the concepts that form the foundation of my horsemanship philosophy. Here, I want to provide a few practical skills that can help you use Horse Speak on your own.

These include:

1. How to Find Zero (p. 37)

2. How to See What Is There (p. 38)

3. Breath Messages (p. 40)

4. The 13 Buttons (p. 41)

5. The Four Gs (p. 45)

6. Healthy Touch (p. 46)

7. The Essence of Liberty Work (p. 49)

Having a basic understanding of these seven keys will also give you a source of reference as you read the stories ahead and greater clarity as I describe the ways Horse Speak solves problems between horses and humans.

How to Find Zero

To find your Zero, the state of inner calm I've mentioned as being the goal and starting place for all your work with your horse, try these tips:

- Think about a beautiful moment.

- Think about a favorite song.

- Take deep breaths.

- Massage your eye muscles.

- Massage your breastbone.

- Stroke your arms downward, one at a time.

- Bend down and touch your toes for a moment.

- Tell your horse, out loud, whatever is stressing you out. Note: Your horse should be loose in his stall or pen when you do this. Do not touch him while you talk. Pat or touch him only after you feel less anxious.

The main idea of getting to Zero is to tell your body that you are safe; your body can relax. The limbic system is responsible for you feeling tense or calm, and it does not respond to reason. Our world tends to be so stressful that our bodies can get "stuck" in a state of low-level hyper-vigilance. This shows up in your face (massage your eye muscles), in your breathing (massage your sternum), and in your overall body tension (stroke your arms). Yoga or Tai Chi or painting or journaling are all other ways to de-stress *before* you get to your horse.

Finding Zero for yourself means you will be able to help your horse find his true Zero, as well.

How to See What Is There

When we first begin to observe horses, we may get stuck in the idea that they are "just eating hay" or "just standing around" or "just swishing at flies." Well, as soon as you hear yourself say "just" anything, that is a clue that *something* is happening "just" beyond your level of awareness.

There are a few ways to enjoy the art of observation and trick yourself into seeing what is really happening:

- Copycat a horse's movements—do what he does—and see if he does them back. This can be a kind of game between you and the horse.

- Mimic his motions—make the faces he makes, turn, walk, and stop when he does. You can do this even some distance away, as it is just an opportunity for you to gain awareness.

- Try one relaxed "O" posture and wait three minutes to see what the horse does (when horses are thinking, time can pass extremely slowly…)

- From outside the fence, make a big "X" posture and see what he does (again allow the horse time to think).

- Count how many motions your horse repeats.

- Ask yourself good questions: How often does your horse look at a certain area, lower his head, raise his head, and so on.

The next step is to pay attention to your approach to the horse. Wait *outside* the horse's enclosure, and literally kick a few boards along the fence line or on neighboring stalls. This may sound funny to do, but Mother horses secure the environment for their babies, and later Lead horses perform this action for the herd. Once you have "secured the environment," begin your approach to your horse, watching for a soft, welcoming expression in his face. If he appears to stiffen up or leans away from you as though he wants to leave, you have touched the edge of his "bubble of personal space." Pause and wait or even back up. If he looks softly toward you, however, even if he is grazing and simply leans his muzzle in your direction, you have a green light to come closer. Most of us get confused at first between a horse who is deferring space (which is a soft respectful sign) and a horse's "X" posture (a horse is declining to engage you). This is an excellent way to train your eye to notice the difference in the feel and the expression of your horse. The *approach and retreat* process is *very* important to horses. They ask permission to enter each other's personal space. When you pay attention to their personal space they will pay more attention to you, and end up desiring to share space with you. If you are patient and wait until a horse seems to soften up before resuming your approach, the horse will be more respectful and relaxed with you.

As we discussed in the last chapter, when it comes to expression and what the horse is "saying," there are many variables to the horse's ears alone (see p. 32). If you are not sure what the face of your horse is "saying," then copy it! For example, we both have highly flexible lips and use them for a wide variety of expressions. Horse facial expressions mirror ours to a certain extent, or vice versa, so try to make the same face as your horse, and you will get a sense of what he is feeling on a certain level. However, try not to label that feeling right away because it will likely be more about what you are feeling than what the horse is feeling (we tend to think horses are out to get us for some reason). Strive to see what is happening from the horse's perspective; see if you can discover what would be making him feel that way and make that face.

Observing is the first part, and interpretation is second. We can't help ourselves: we interpret things all the time, but we usually assign meaning to things a little too quickly. The trick to interpreting Horse Speak is to stay curious and open. I like to use a catch phrase like, "How interesting," or "How curious," or "I wonder what that could be?"

Even if you have no idea what a horse means by his body language, the simple fact that you are observing him while at the state of Zero communicates your intention to get to know him better.

Breath Messages

Out of necessity, horses need to stay as "quiet" as possible (inside and out) to not attract predators. They utilize their breathing to create a whole platform of communication through subtle sounds. Really explaining how we can do breath messages is not possible in a book (you need to hear and see them to truly understand them—my DVD *Horse Speak: First Conversations* helps clarify many breath messages). In the meantime, here are a few helpful hints.

- We should copy soft, sniffing, "curious" breaths when we want to smell something nice. This "Interested Breath" is also the breath horses use to say they are curious about something or about you.

- Strong, blowing out breaths—as though you were blowing out candles—mimics the sound horses make when they announce a potential threat. I call this "Sentry Breath" or "blowing away the bogeyman."

- Two rapid inhales and one long exhale mimics the horse's "Shuddering Breath," which is used to say, "All's clear; I am feeling better; we are feeling better; let's feel better."

- A short snort, sounding like a little piggy snort, is used by mares with their foals. This "Nurturing Breath" signals a soft, nurturing moment.

- Deep breathing (focus on your floating ribs, moving your entire rib cage), what I call "Deliberate Breathing," signals that all is well, and it is time to release any leftover tension.

- Soft, huffing breaths into or aimed toward a horse's muzzle (even at a distance—do not put your face up to a horse you don't know) signals interest, friendliness, and connection. This is the "Greeting Breath."

As with copying facial expressions, when you notice your horse breathing in a particular way, you may want to mimic him. At the very least, this will help you understand what sort of breathing your horse likes in certain situations.

The 13 Buttons

To make Horse Speak a little easier for us to grasp, I have reduced key equine communication points to the 13 most prevalent places or "Buttons," as I call them (see illustration on p. 42). The horse's body has many Buttons and sub-Buttons, but these 13 centers of discourse offer the most direct conversation points and are the easiest to find and work with.

The Buttons can activate a horse to move in some way or hold him in place (like a version of "Stay!" for a dog, although with horses it usually means "Stay with me" and is a sign of bonding and connectedness). You can activate a horse to move away from you or to stop doing what he is doing or to change direction or back up—or you can activate a Button to ask him to come toward you by using a beckoning message. Each Button has a specific meaning attached to it, but it is also true that horses have different emotional responses to their Buttons, depending on what has happened to them. Any Button can be asked to *hold still, move away*, or *come toward*, although certain Buttons tend to be used in specific situations. Over time you can acquire a deeper understanding of the Buttons and the nuances of the language they communicate. The Buttons are centers for meaning, and associations and inferences related to them are very personal to our horses.

In my book *Horse Speak*, and in my DVD by the same name, I go into great detail when it comes to the 13 Buttons and their effects. Here are a few key ideas about activating or holding a Button:

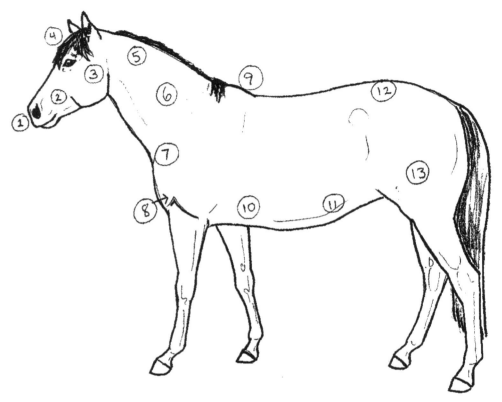

1 Greeting Button

2 Play Button

3 Go Away Face Button

4 Friendly Button

5 Follow Me Button

6 Mid-Neck Button

7 Shoulder Button

8 Back-Up Button

9 Grooming Button

10 Girth Button

11 Jump-Up Button

12 Hip-Drive Button

13 Yield-Over Button

- *Activate Away or Sending Message*: Placing your pointer finger on or aiming it at a Button—even just holding it up in the air toward one—tells a horse you desire to activate (move). The secret is to hold it there for a *long* moment—do not shake or wave your hand in the air. Think of how many times you have seen one horse drive another away simply by using one *long* "stare-down." Occasionally, a horse may use a mild head toss to emphasize his feelings, but the more powerful the horse, the less movement he wants to use to get his message through.

- *Activate Come Back or Beckoning Message*: Aiming your pointer finger and then scooping it toward yourself as you back up a few steps in your "O" posture signals you want your horse to come toward you. This is just like the "Come here" finger curl we use with other people, only as you scoop your finger toward yourself, make a motion that resembles pulling threads off the Button you are activating and into your lap. This "pulling sensation" triggers a desire in the horse to want to come to you. Try it with friends!

- *Stay Still*: Holding your palm against a Button tells the horse to either hold still while *in connection* with you or to push back toward you and come to you.

- *Sniffing a Button* tells the horse you won't harm him in that place; you are buddies. (With horses, this is most often seen around the neck, but they will also sniff each other's bellies and rumps...you may not want to sniff that far!)

- *Touching the Girth Button* with your palm asks the horse to "line up"—imagine a marching band getting ready to go. It again needs to be noted that horses are very subtle; there is a difference between "buddying up" at the Shoulder Button (see p. 44), which implies rest (or even a nap!), and "lining up" at the Girth Button in a state of readiness like you might see in two driving horses yoked together. The touch on the Girth Button can be in preparation to go somewhere, or to hold steady right where you are. Think of how horses "go somewhere" together: Pals can line up with each other at the girth, but horses that are not friends won't do this. When a horse moves carefully and slowly past you, I call it a "Sail-By"—he is "showing" you the Girth Button (as well as all the rest of his buttons) and is saying he is open to connecting with you. Horses intend to go somewhere together when they initiate communication with this Button. However, they can also ask for space by aiming a message here, which typically results in the receiving horse moving off sideways or forward. Foals line up with their heads aimed here to keep in stride with Mom. Since this Button is pretty much in the center of the horse's rib cage, breath messages can influence it a great deal. When riding, our legs and heels are sending quite a lot of information to this area. It is a good idea to explore as many conversations as possible with this Button because we use it so much.

- *Touching the Shoulder Button* has multiple meanings, as well. If you are seeking to establish yourself as a Leader for your horse, then you can use the Shoulder Button (in conjunction with either the Mid-Neck or Go Away Face Button) to request the horse give you more room or step aside. Since all hierarchical conversations between horses deal with the core value of "personal space," this Button is very efficient in gently demonstrating that you "own" the space. However, the Shoulder Button can also ask a horse to "buddy up" with you. This is not as serious as the "line up" request at the Girth Button, which implies more of a need to stick together. "Buddy up" says, "We are pals, we can hang out," or "Let's take a nap." Placing your palm on the Shoulder Button and remaining still, or simply standing at the shoulder without touching him, tells a horse you want to share space. Since horses do not spend a lot of time touching each other, standing quietly near each other is an important part of social connection. Hint: Horses prefer us to stand closer to the Shoulder Button. Standing by their heads feels invasive to them, just like it would to us. Picture someone saying hello to you, and shaking your hand, but then never backing up! You would feel crowded and invaded, too.

- *Touching the Hip-Drive Button* sends a "weaker" horse forward and implies the other horse "has his back" (or in other words will kick the coyotes if they come up from behind). Horses use a good deal of gentle touch here: they will sniff, rub their chins or faces on the Button, or use their "X" expression to send a nervous horse forward. In disputes, a horse may get bitten in this area, as well—a dominant horse may seem to forcefully drive a timid horse forward from this Button. But in most situations, there is one big outrush of intensity, and then it is over. Note: We must be very careful with this Button. I advise asking for simple steps forward or sideways, one at a time, to simulate the kind, patient rearranging a Mentor horse will do when telling a timid horse he "has his back." Use both a palm-down gesture and your pointer finger to see what your horse says about it. *Always use caution, however.* If the horse tucks his tail, hunches down, throws his head up, or demonstrates any other "X" messages, only try activating or holding this Button from over a stall wall or fence. Your horse will still see it. I have had a horse up to 50 feet away respond to activation of this Button. You are only looking for a flinch, a lean, or a single step at first. The less you ask for in the beginning, the more willing your horse will become to move off easily and without tension or resistance later on.

When working with the 13 Buttons remember that horses thrive on rhythmic *anything*. Rhythm is the theme of their lives. We ride them because the rhythm of their gaits feels so good to us! There is a rhythm to using Horse Speak, as well.

The Four Gs

I call the four primary "stages" of Horse Speak the "Four Gs." They include:

1. *Greeting*: The stage when you initiate contact, attend to a protocol of politeness, sort out hierarchy/leadership roles, and establish "special needs" by determining how near or far apart you should be. A careful touch of muzzle to muzzle or knuckles (human) to muzzle is used as a respectful offering to communicate. Both the Greeting Button and Go Away Face Button can be employed during this stage.

2. *Going Somewhere*: This initiates leader/follower protocol, includes making space on all sides (in front, behind, side to side), and requests a horse follow the leader. This stage can be completed in one moment or take all day. It occurs in two

When activating or holding a Button, leave your hand in the air for *one full minute*. Horses *react* quickly and on pure instinct, but they *think* very slowly and all the way through. You may get your answer a full minute after you ask something! That's right—just stand there and wait. Horses are not machines or computers. You cannot push a button and get a response that is authentic in a matter of seconds. In fact, if a horse is rushing to answer you, he is not thinking it all the way through and may be worried about upsetting you instead.

parts: First there is awareness of the intention of movement and the Buttons in play while *not* trying to walk anywhere (best used in a stall, paddock, or pen). Second, you actually move off together, sorting out who moves whom, and how to make turns, stops, and starts together. Going Somewhere mimics the ability of a herd to move cohesively.

3. *Grooming* can be the hardest of the four stages of Horse Speak to authentically reach because horses do not initiate deeper levels of connection until the Greeting and Going Somewhere rituals are satisfied. Grooming initiates *all* forms on intimacy (including contact and distance intimacy), uses beckoning and balancing gestures (balanced horses are relaxed), uses "O" postures, and includes any affection, connection, or deeper relaxation.

4. *Gone* is the end of the discussion. When a horse swishes his tail at someone, he is saying the moment—whatever kind of moment it might be—is over. This also includes a version of "No": shaking the tail and stomping a foot when the horse is asked to do something he does not want to do. In stronger examples, "No" can be accompanied by a squeal or a strike.

Understanding what the Four Gs look like and how to navigate them is integral to being able to communicate and connect with your horse.

Healthy Touch

A great deal of Horse Speak is achieved by, at first, *not* touching your horse. Horses are not dogs and do not actually enjoy "rough" up-and-down petting or having their faces grabbed and smooched. As I've said, they value space more than touch. Touch in the herd only occurs after the environment is known to be secure, the herd is at rest, and all is well. But because they live with humans who have hands and love to use them, most horses have learned to adapt to our need to touch them. We value the sensation of touch with our animals.

Horses do enjoy being touched, but only after it has been offered at the right time and place, and only when we link it to positive feelings the horse is also experiencing. In this way, touch reinforces positive feedback. The wrong kind of touch, too much touch, and forced touch can cause a horse to shut down because he has been taught he cannot refuse.

There are any number of fabulous programs that provide options for "healthy" and respectful ways to touch your horse, for example Linda Telling-ton-Jones's Tellington Method; Jim Masterson's Masterson Method; Margret Henkels's Conformation Balancing; therapeutic massage; and Reiki, just to name a few. In addition, I have a few simple tricks and tips to help you clue into what "healthy touch" feels like for horses.

In 2016, David Linden, author of *Touch: The Science of the Hand, Heart, and Mind* (Penguin Books, 2016), gave a TED Talk about the science of touch that you can easily find via Google. He is funny and fascinating throughout, but one thing stood out to me that I want to paraphrase here: It turns out that we are hard-wired to *tune out* the sensations we experience *internally*, and our brains instead favor input from *outside* ourselves. Linden states that this ensures we get our needs met by paying attention to the world around us. He also explains that we feel touch differently when someone else initiates it versus when we touch ourselves.

This filled in some blanks for me when it came to why healthy touch is so important to learn when it comes to interactions between horses and humans. When we are in our "tuned-out" state, we can end up mindlessly touching our horses. We are not empathically linked to whether *they* are emotionally enjoying our touch, but *we* are enjoying the sensation of touching them, so too often we think they like what we are doing, too.

A horse might enjoy some aspects of the *physical* act of getting a scratch but not be *emotionally* fulfilled by that action at all. You will see this horse either start rubbing as mindlessly and emphatically on the person as she is on him, giving back the same sensation he has learned to tolerate, or start pulling away and dancing around, seeking to end the contact.

To initiate healthy touch with your horse:

- At all times use rhythm, firm but not hard contact, and consistent speed—not too fast, not too slow.

- Begin by making contact at the withers. Horses usually start here with each other, so you are at least broadcasting your intention.

- Stroke downward at the "Friendly Button" (see p. 42) on the top of the horse's head between the eyes if he will allow it. This is the sec-ond-most-used contact spot between horses.

- Stroke over and around the horse's eyes with a soft downward caress. Most horses come to crave this touch in time. (Imagine not being able to rub your own eyes when you need to, unless you lean over and do it against your knee or on a fence?)

- Use your hand in a downward motion when stroking. Horses' hair grows "downhill"; they do not really like us to go "against the grain" (this is similar with cats).

- Attempt to scratch the throat and chest of your horse. I find they usually really enjoy this.

- Make small, circular motions with your hand. If you watch horses groom each other, they make rhythmic, circular motions with their teeth.

- Inhale audibly with your face near your horse's body as you scratch or stroke him. Horses sniff each other when they feel connected.

- Try an action called "cupping": Shape your hand into a cup as though holding water in your palm. Pat rhythmically and firmly along the topline of the horse. This can help muscle release. (In Swedish massage this is one of the types of tapotement—a technique of rapid and repeated striking of the body—used.)

- Hold, cup, and scratch areas of the rump if you can. Horses find this soothing.

- Avoid releasing your tension into your horse by touching him when you feel nervous.

- Also avoid touching him when *he* seems nervous, unless you have a specific form of touch that you and your horse both agree is soothing. Otherwise, you may be overstimulating your horse at a time when he is already hyper-vigilant.

- Use deep breathing and a subtle rocking motion from your body to his as often as you can to signal that you want your touch to feel emotionally soothing.

- If at any time your horse "shivers" when you touch him, this indicates inner tension. Seek ways to help him find Zero.

- If your horse shows no reaction or response to your touch at all, he may be "shut down." Go through all the Buttons (see p. 42) until you find one spot that lets you make contact.(see p. 42)

The bottom line is that most horses actually do enjoy some level of touching and being touched. I have met quite a few terrified animals that learned to love and even crave physical affection over time. Some horses seem to be pushy about touch and may rub on us too hard with their heads, or demand we scratch them. Even when this is the case, I have found more often than not that a pushy horse is still reacting to feeling invaded—it's just that he took the proverbial bull by the horns and is saying, "Oh, yeah? If humans are going to always walk right up to me, then I am going to do it to them, too!"

Horses are more similar to us than we think, in that we are very specific about who gets to touch us and how and when. Some people love massage, while others hate it. Some people are super-huggy-bears, while others would rather hide than embrace. Horses are all unique and will love touch more or less depending on their character. We mustn't be afraid to touch our horses; I simply suggest that we give them the right to take a breath and feel ready for that level of intimacy. It is as important to them as it is to us.

The Essence of Liberty Work

Liberty work is very alluring because it implies a deeper relationship between horse and handler, since the horse is responding to requests while "free." It certainly can be inspiring to watch a master at liberty work moving in harmony with one or even several loose horses.

However, there is a common belief when practicing and performing liberty work that the horse must move off at a trot or canter for the conversation to begin. This is not the case.

Because my work over the years has involved so many rescue horses that could not be moved out in such a way, whether due to injuries, the after-effects of starvation, or issues of abuse, I had to whittle away at the core conversations we can have at liberty. I realized that by using what I call the "Reverse Round Pen"—in which I ask the horse to *not move at all*, but stay where he is as I move around him—I could find the "edge" of the horse's comfort zone and where he would begin to desire to move away from the pressure of my presence. If I was sensitive to this, *I* could move away from him, allowing him to stay put and begin to understand that I respected his space and his emotional state. This ultimately became very useful and successful in my work. It allowed horses to initiate conversations with me in which we gradually built trust and mutual respect, simply because I behaved like a Mother, a Leader, or a Mentor who said, "You're hurt; don't move."

In one dramatic case, a rescue horse had gotten her foot stuck in a fence and severely injured her ankle. She was limping around out in the field but would not let anyone catch her. I "Reverse Round-Penned" her until she became very calm, which allowed me to approach, halter, and lead her back to the stall for treatment.

Try "skating" on the outside of the horse's "bubble of personal space." Find the edge of it and linger there as you attempt to make a complete circle around him. If he starts to flinch you have gone too far. When he uses his "O" posture to gaze toward you—even if he is just keeping an ear on you—then you are skating the edge of his bubble. This will inform you both about your inner level of Zero, and your outer "X" and "O," as well as your horse's Zero, "X," and "O." One reason this is so important is because the 13 Buttons (see p. 42) all have different contact points. If your core energy is aiming at a Button and you don't realize it, you may tell your horse something you didn't mean to. By circling the horse and making the game about *not* moving him, you will experience changes in both your feelings of awareness and his.

As I touched on earlier, horses often do what I call a "Sail-By" with us: they saunter very slowly past us and then make a circle or arc to saunter back to us or even just position themselves so that we can see all their Buttons. This is their way of opening up conversation. It's like they're saying, "Hey there! Here are all of my Buttons. What do you want to talk about?" When you do the Reverse Round Pen, you are simulating this act. You are saying, "Hey there! Let me see if I can talk to all your Buttons." And you are doing it at an extremely slow speed, which makes your likelihood of success higher. One of the dangers of sending a horse out to trot or canter around you, whether on a longe line or in a round pen, is that you have to control which Button you are aiming at, how you are aiming, and what level of intensity is appropriate to use, all while the horse is moving very fast. This is a fast-paced conversation in which nuance still matters a great deal. If you get "out of position" even for a moment, you may think you are saying something when in reality you are telling your horse something completely different.

Having worked with hundreds of rescue horses through the years, poor longeing and round-penning techniques are a pet peeve. I feel they make rehabilitation of a horse that much harder. I am *not* saying these tools do not have a place; in fact, they can provide some very important lessons in a horse's education. What I *am* saying is that the feel, timing, care, self-awareness, and sensitivity of the horse's experience is something that has to be carefully culti-vated. Why risk losing ground by going too fast? Start slow and build up, just like everything else we have ever learned. We don't begin with calculus; we begin with basic numbers. And Zero is one of them.

Keeping your Zero and helping your horse keep his will set you up to have engaging play, at any speed. So...easy does it.

I believe that liberty work using Horse Speak opens whole new worlds of possibilities about having conversations under any circumstances, not just when big things are happening. Liberty means just that: *freedom*. If a horse is free, then he must also be free to choose to engage...or not. Asking a horse to move off to *initiate* conversation is like telling a friend that we can only talk if we go jogging. I think most of us agree that a quiet conversation over a cup of tea is often preferable to trying to jog and share anything meaningful. Of course, when we have a good friendship, we may enjoy many different sce-narios in each other's company: going for a hike or skiing or swimming, going shopping or out to dinner, or just sitting quietly together. There are different levels of sharing that take place in a quality friendship; this needs to be the case in the friendship we have with our horses, as well.

The Reverse Round Pen is a way for me to find Zero for myself and for the horse I'm connecting with. As you read the stories ahead, look for the moments when I talk about pausing, backing up, and approaching a horse differently. The goal of this concept is to have your horse *not* move away from you. So often, we approach our horses and send them out to run, thinking this is the only way to begin communicating. The truth is, they were communicat-ing with us from the moment they saw us.

Part Two

true stories

Chapter 4

My Horses, My Teachers

I didn't know I was shopping for a horse.

I was traveling home from my sister's house, a good three-hour drive, when I pulled off the highway to get a bite to eat. I happened to pass a horse ranch called Happy Acres and noticed a sign announcing an "open house." I thought about this all during lunch, and on my way back down the road to the highway, I decided to stop in—even though it was late February, and I had a bum knee at the time and was using a cane.

Curious-er and Curious-er

Hobbling over to the visitor gift shop, I learned that this farm not only rescued horses but also worked with kids with special needs. Several of their students were on hand to offer a beaming smile and a friendly "walk around." I was escorted by Paul, a 14-year-old student with some physical and learning handicaps who nonetheless got around just fine. He was chatty and happy and loved these horses with all his heart.

He asked me what I did to my knee, and I replied I had slipped on some ice that winter. He gleefully told me to wear good boots.

Then, into the barn aisle strode a tall man who moved fast for someone who "had molasses on his boots." At first glance, he seemed to be in slow motion, but all at once, he was standing in front of me. It reminded me of an old Buddhist saying: "Hurry slowly."

It turned out that he was the owner of this farm, a fellow named Doug, and he particularly loved Appaloosas and Paints and rode Western. He was a kind man who took in as many "lil' orphans" as he could—which included pot-bellied pigs, an emu, goats, and even a half-zebra-half-pony known as "Ziny." All the animals issued an air of calm, even though the place was quite crowded.

Doug told me he regularly traveled out West to Appaloosa and Paint breeding ranches and scooped up the yearlings to train for sale as 4-H prospects. Some of his horses were quite talented and did well in shows.

When we broached the topic of training methodology, Doug seemed open-minded about what he termed the "New Age horsemanship stuff" that was growing in popularity. His down-home horse wisdom told him that people were just trying to find another way to "get there," and if nobody got hurt, he didn't mind the newfound interest in horses that came along with it.

I enjoyed talking to Doug; he was a man of few words but well-chosen ones. He had a ready smile and seemed at peace surrounded by his students and animals.

I had been working with a friend's horses, having recently relocated to Vermont, so I tried to pick his brain about some of the problems we were having. I had been busy raising my family and my return to my horse passion was only recent as my kids became older and I had more free time.

Seemingly out of nowhere, Doug told me to wait right where I was. I sat on a mounting block in the indoor arena while he fetched one of his new "prospects."

Sister Golden Hair Surprise

In walked a honey dun, snowflake Appaloosa with hazel green eyes and black eyelids, which made it look as if she was wearing eyeliner. Not only was she a soft, golden color, but her undercoat was dappled, and there were zebra stripes on her chestnut legs. I didn't know what hit me.

Doug had her saddled up and told me to go ahead and get on the mare. I questioned the suggestion, reminding him of my bad knee with the brace on it. He told me to ride without stirrups as though it was silly to even ask.

The moment I sat in the rather large saddle, I "heard" this horse "say," "Well, what do you want?"

In all my previous years of riding, I had never had this experience. Not knowing what to do, I told Doug what I thought I'd heard. He just grinned from ear to ear and said that he had a feeling that would happen. He indicated I should ask the mare, who he called Dakota, to go out on the rail at a walk.

As I settled into her light steps, Doug told me that this was his special horse—one that he was thinking of keeping for himself. Although she was only two years old, she was brighter than most and had some big opinions of herself to go along with it. He said that occasionally a horse comes along who "sees right through you and your garbage, and makes you dig a little deeper." Dakota was such a horse.

Doug said that the way I was feeling on Dakota's back was the way *all* horses should feel when I swung up onto them. They should have their own mind, and yet they should not be closed to yours. He told me to memorize what I was feeling and try to recreate it with the horses I was working with back home.

I only rode Dakota for about five minutes, but it changed me forever.

Dreams and Reality

I went back to Happy Acres several times to visit and volunteer with Doug's programs, although it was over an hour away from my home. Each time, I would linger with Dakota and try to understand what was different about her and why my perception shifted when I was near her.

Then one day Doug told me he had to sell off a bunch of horses because he was bringing in about 35 pregnant mares he had rescued from a roundup. He asked if I wanted Dakota.

The opportunity was not something I could pass up. I scrambled the money together and hastily decided for her to live with a friend of mine, who had a barn down the road from my home, seeing as I didn't have a paddock or shelter in my backyard.

One last late season snowstorm had blown through a week before I went to pick up Dakota. I asked the barn staff to bring her in for me because there was so much ice everywhere, and I was afraid for my knee. Waiting on the other side of the indoor ring as my new horse was led toward me, I was shocked to see her rear straight up—and walk several steps on her hind legs!—while the handler paid her no mind and just kept on walking.

Slack-jawed, I asked him to turn her loose in the indoor because she clearly needed to let off some steam. He smiled and did just that, and I witnessed some acrobatics I had never seen before.

Oh, my.

He noticed my pale face and laughingly told me, "Ah, she is harmless. She just likes to show off."

A few other boarders were nearby, and they asked me what I was doing with Dakota. I told them I had just bought her. They flatly stated I had better have double locks on everything because she was notorious for getting loose and letting everyone else in the barn out, to boot.

Oh, dear.

Doug showed up just as Dakota finally rolled and stood up, shaking it all off. He chuckled and said, "You want to know what makes a horse tick? She'll show you. Don't worry about it, she wouldn't hurt a fly."

Nodding his hat to me, and with a little twinkle in his eye, he left.

Oh, crap.

Good, Bad, and Surprise

Dakota seemed to settle into her new life with me very quickly. My teenage daughter Amber had been taking riding lessons for some time, so I asked her to get on "Kota," as we called her, while I watched. I needed to see the "action" from the ground.

They moved off together like they were old friends. My daughter smiled and thanked me for buying us a horse. It was a dream-come-true moment.

Then the saddle slipped.

I was not used to knot-tying on Western rigging, and I knew instantly I had not tightened it enough. Amber was caught off guard and tried to cling to the mare's neck. Kota scooted forward a few steps as the whole kit and caboodle slipped down her side. My daughter was planted butt-first on the ground.

"Ouch!" she cried out as the pain and embarrassment hit her at the same time. In this major Bad-Mom Moment, I didn't know whether to run to my daughter first or to try to catch the horse, dragging the saddle under her belly.

I chose to get my kid out of harm's way, as I had no way of knowing how Kota would react to this situation. Amber limped over to the mounting block to sit down, gingerly, on her bruised bottom. I tried to soothe her as she yelled at me through tears.

Time passes differently in a crisis. Just as I settled Amber onto the mounting block and was turning to deal with what I was certain might have become a bucking bronc show, I realized that Kota had followed us to where we were, dragging the saddle along upside-down, as though she carried it that way every day.

Looking up from my squatting position, I noticed that her ears were sideways and her eyes were tented. To me, this looked like real concern. I had been in dozens of horse accidents, including having a horse flip over with me when he caught his front legs on a jump. What I was accustomed to occurring was for the horse to wander off or even run away.

This was not the case, though. Kota was not only standing protectively over Amber, she began to lick her helmet, like a mother lion might lick her cub. Amber had been riding since she was nine, and she'd also had her fair share of accidents. We were both shocked into silence.

With wide eyes, my daughter asked, "Is she *licking* me?"

I nodded my head, and Amber forgot all about her pain as she stood up to hug Kota around her neck. I jumped up to untangle the saddle, and then we all just hung out in the ring together…and started to really get to know each other.

Horse of a Different Color

Amber became an avid bareback rider after this event. She practiced vaulting off the ever-patient Kota and mounting from strange places. With my daughter, Kota seemed to feel a sort of sisterhood. As a young mare, it seemed she could relate.

With me, it was a different story. There was some sort of super-intelligence in this horse that baffled me, and I was drawn to try many of the modern "horse whispering" techniques that my clinic addiction at the time was instilling in me.

Kota was a gentle, kind soul on one hand—and on the other she was a fire-breathing dragon. She enjoyed trail riding with gusto and jumped anything in her path. She still loved to rear and could buck in place several times in a row without ever putting tension into the lead rope. She was an acrobatically inclined athlete. I knew that without developing her mind to the fullest, this mare could become dangerous if she ever soured.

Then, only six months after I bought her, Kota was injured when a stick impaled her leg. We never knew how she did it—the vet guessed she was fooling around in the field and landed just the right way on just the right object (the way horses sometimes do). I was told she would be on stall rest for about three months, so I hurried to finish the paddock in my backyard and arranged to bring her home.

Angels and Devils

Kota seemed to fit right in at our place. With her leg bandaged, she couldn't move around very quickly or well. We were supposed to hand-walk her twice a day and keep her secured in her large run-in shelter the rest of the time. Her prognosis was in question: the vet was not sure how sound she would be when the wound healed.

I had to change Kota's bandage and give her injections twice a day. The vet bills were mounting and the stress of tending to her needs was making me rethink the whole adventure. Doug had told me that if anything at all came up, to send Dakota back to him and not sell her off to the world. It was a dark moment for me.

I got up in the early dawn one morning to have a cup of coffee out back with Kota and try to think about what I should do. As I rounded the corner of my house, the morning mist that is so common mid-July in Vermont was rising to the treetops around the edge of her paddock. We had staked out a 12-foot enclosure in front of her shelter so she could move around a bit more, and she was standing there, under the trees with her front feet up on a stump we had left in her paddock. She often liked to stand that way. We called it "Proud Kota Stump."

A light breeze toyed with her mane and at that exact moment, the sun poked through the trees and the mist, cascading rays of light like you see in paintings of God or the saints down onto my horse.

All that was missing was the singing of angels.

"Okay, okay, okay!" I said to the world. "I get it!"

Kota looked at me—and then looked right through me. She had done this before, but under the influence of this amazing scene, I felt myself tear up and let go. Going to her, I placed my forehead on her neck and vowed that no matter what, I was there to learn, and my skin was in the game.

Solid Gold

The golden mare in my backyard was forcing me to dig deeper, just like Doug said she would. Since all the natural-horsemanship-type work I'd learned involved running around in round pens or on long lead lines, and my horse was not supposed to do more than walk a little bit, I needed new tools to connect with her.

I returned to something I had learned long ago.

Growing up, I had been fortunate to ride a Fourth-Level dressage horse during lessons because my riding teacher had trained at the Spanish Riding School and believed it was how I would learn. I was the lucky recipient of her new-world-view of horsemanship and was groomed as a protégé. I helped with some green horses, learning a great deal about longeing and in-hand techniques. But just when I was really rounding a corner in my education as a rider and trainer, I fell in love, got married, and ended my "hobby" to raise my kids.

My love for animals transferred to dogs, and I became a dog trainer. My love for learning took me to night classes as I got my degree in art. Having suffered my whole life from severe asthma, I also pursued an interest in meditation, yoga, and Reiki to try to heal myself. I became a Reiki practitioner and teacher while my kids were small, because I could set my own hours, and I felt I was doing some kind of good in the world. Eventually, martial arts and modern dance became a way to not only still my inner self but strengthen my body, as well. Always seeking new paths toward physical health and well-being, I sought the help of a medicine man, who took me under his wing and taught me many things about working in harmony with nature.

Each of these pursuits required intense patience, inner mindfulness, openness, and awareness of details. And with Dakota, all those years dedicated to learning very nuanced and detailed things about body, mind, and spirit would find a new outlet. While she was on stall rest, she needed me to rethink everything I ever thought I knew about working with horses. It was not possible to longe her or work with her in the round pen. In fact, all she could do at first was limp a few steps here and there.

What could I do to help us move forward? I started by digging up anything and everything I could on classical dressage—my roots—including several books written at the turn of the century.

Slowly, I began to adapt the in-hand techniques I'd begun to learn from my instructor all those years before to our needs.

The Rabbit Hole

With Kota and I enjoying such interesting sessions, I wanted to learn more about what sort of thoughtful mind games we could play.

I ventured into clicker training to learn about the feel and timing that many marine mammal trainers have. After all, if you can train an aquatic animal to do tricks without using ropes or whips, what could similar techniques do for a horse?

I learned quite a bit about shaping behaviors and found the work to be very engaging. However, when I tried to bring what I was learning to the riding school where I was now working, I was not met with enthusiasm. The barn owner did not want lesson horses searching for treats from students; she felt it was a liability. Nor was she interested in using natural horsemanship methods, because she ran what she considered an "English" riding school and felt that would be confusing for students.

So I decided to figure out how to use the same feel and timing of mindful connection that I had cultivated during my hand-walking sessions with Dakota with the school horses to see if I could help them become happier in their work *without* using treats. I wanted to be able to build rapport between horses and students so that their time together was as positive for the horses as it was for the people.

I had become aware of the importance of *pausing*. In clicker training, there is a moment when you pause and deliver the treat. This shows the "game" is over, and everyone has a moment to recover. In natural horsemanship, there is the idea that you only ask until you get a "try," and then you quit asking like a hot potato. You pause. This creates lightness.

Hmmmmm.

Both worlds used pausing or quitting to signal, "Yes," to the horse. So I thought that maybe my best first step would be teaching my students to look for the smallest "try" in everything so they would know when to pause. And what would the praise be, since I couldn't treat the school horses? I thought again about my work with Dakota and how we communicated with each other. We often breathed with each other in a moment of rest. So I began taking a breath during a pause after a "try" to reward the horses.

This had amazing results. In only a few weeks, the horses were more relaxed, and the students felt they had more of a rapport with them. The sour horses became softer and the nervous horses became braver.

I began to bring other lessons from Dakota into the school and started to teach the students to become aware of *how* their horses walked while on the lead rope, not just where their heads were. I began riding lessons on the ground, with cones to weave in and out of and ground poles to step over, so each horse-and-rider pair could practice being "in step" with each other.

AHA MOMENT

I discovered that if I focused on each balanced footstep Dakota took when I hand-walked her and whether her movement arose from her own core and "pivot point" (the center around which she rotated), our time together turned into something similar to Tai Chi for the horse. Step by step we made our way into all sorts of lateral work. Kota's love for learning meant that each new session drove both of us into a shared experience of a "dance" we were making up together. She began to offer ideas and suggestions, and I could mimic her and find my own corresponding movements.

In Tai Chi there is an exercise called "push hands." This calls for both participants to place their wrists together and move in connection with each other as one pushes against the other. The goal is not to push anyone over but to learn to bend with the energy of the "opponent" and effectively take the wind out of his or her sails. I was finding a sort of "push hands" with Dakota as we learned to pivot and move around and with each other. Since I did this while taking her for her daily walk, we also had to move in straight lines.

In some dressage manuals, I discovered the saying, "Shoulder-in fixes everything." Shoulder-in is one lateral movement performed both in-hand and under saddle, although most people do it while riding. Since schools of different thought offered various opinions on how best to achieve this movement, Dakota and I simply enjoyed the spirit of exploration. She could move in amazing ways—as I mentioned, she was an acrobat—and she could easily rebalance herself into some new move she made up. Together, we found what kind of gymnastic exercise worked for us.

More importantly, I got to learn about how, when, and where to hold all *my* body parts to either flow along with her, or lead the dance.

By the time the vet said her leg was healed, she was in great physical shape, and ready to ride.

Eventually, I started asking the students and horses to create a little lateral movement or even just awareness of the horse standing or moving in balance, both on the ground and during their warm up and cool down.

The effect was amazing. Horses not only became more compliant and willing, but the students felt like their riding was becoming less forced, more natural, and more "happy."

Yes, everyone felt happy.

I suddenly realized that much of the riding I had done as a student myself was *not* happy— interesting, addicting, and sometimes it really felt good…but not always happy.

In a flash of insight, I realized the question Dakota had been asking me all this time wasn't, "What do you want?"

It was, "What do you *really* want?"

LICK AND CHEW

My "low," my darkest moment, was the opportunity for Dakota and me to dig deeper. By realizing what balance meant to my horse, not just what I could get my horse to do with her feet, I was able to reach whole new levels of understanding about what horses are looking for in a human partner and how important their foot placement is to them.

This, combined with more exploration into the "thoughtful" and mindful work that was already available, led me to investigate the more intricate concepts of intimate but powerful approaches to being with horses.

Chapter 5

Silver

One afternoon I got a call from my neighbor asking if I would help her with a new pony she had bought for her youngest child. I had met "Rocky" a few times…and honestly was smitten! He was a silver dun of unknown origin. Even the veterinarian could not tell what breed he really was, although he was fairly certain he had been used as a breeding stallion at one point due to his personality.

My neighbor had bought Rocky thinking he could be used for Western pleasure because she had been told he had done some shows and she had seen pictures of him being ridden in Western tack. But apparently the previous owner (who said her kid outgrew the pony in a few months, which is usually code for "too much horse") had been told he had also been someone's eventing horse, and before that he had been a driving horse for the Amish (and still had his handmade harness to prove it).

Well, my neighbor had sent Rocky the Western pleasure pony off to summer camp with her son, and after three days, he had thrown the instructor several times and jumped the fence to attack the 18-hand Belgian who lived in the pen next door.

Rocky, at all of 13.3 hands, had earned the nickname "Pit Bull Pony."

My neighbor knew I had a reputation for helping "difficult" horses come around, so she thought maybe I could spend some time with Rocky and see what his deal was. By then I knew Dakota needed a horse companion, so I agreed to have Rocky come to my place for a few weeks.

He never left.

Digging Deeper

Rocky was unlike any horse I had ever met. He was not entirely unfriendly, but he did not linger for affection or grooming—from horse or human. He could drag anyone, anytime he chose—not even the chain he came with over his nose entirely stopped him. He was rideable...when he saw fit. He did not "feel" like a domestic horse. This occurred to me repeatedly.

One day, while scrolling around on the Internet, I saw the spitting image of Rocky. I clicked on the photo immediately, thinking perhaps one of his previous owners had posted it, and was taken to the home page that talked about the Tarpan—a prehistoric wild horse that ranged from Southern France and Spain eastward to central Russia. The original wild Tarpan died out in the 1800s due to human population growth. (At that time, the Tarpan was seen as a competitor for farmland.) The last surviving wild Tarpan died in a Ukrainian Game Preserve in 1876.

In the 1930s two German zoologists named Heinz and Lutz Heck believed that the Tarpan could be "bred back"—a natural or human attempt to reassemble the genes of an extinct species. They believed certain domesticated European horses that likely descended from the Tarpan still retained that DNA, and by crossing them with Przewalski stallions, they developed the first modern-day "Tarpan."

In the 1950s and '60s, a few American zoos imported some of the bred-back Tarpans, and it is believed that all Tarpans in North America today are likely descended from those original zoo animals. It suddenly seemed to me, I might very well have one of them.

About a week later, my mother turned up an old picture of me as a little girl. We had lived near a small zoo in Massachusetts that we often visited. In the picture, I was squatting next to a chain link fence (and yes, stretching my hand under the fence-guard), and who was reaching toward me but a Tarpan! There were two in that zoo!

Now it made sense why I was so drawn to little Rocky and all his attitude. Somewhere back in my subconscious I recognized him. If anything ever felt like destiny, this was it.

I began to approach my relationship with Rocky with new insight. He had always "felt" wild to me—not feral, but authentically different from any horse or pony I had ever met. What would it take to earn his trust?

When the Student Is Ready, the Teacher Appears

Rocky would become the number one reason I would finally break through my own limitations and reach beyond how I had been conditioned to think about horses and horse training.

The first week he was with me, he kicked, bit, and bucked. It wasn't that he was ever actually mean—which I know seems hard to believe—because his actions were always an answer to what someone was doing.

My daughter was playing with his lips, like she did with Dakota, and he slowly moved his teeth across her fingers, bit down just enough to make his point, then released her.

My son wanted to "hop on," because Rocky seemed so docile when he was standing around in his paddock. Rocky moved at a brisk walk over to the electric fence, dropped his shoulder and gave just enough of a buck to dump Josh right onto it.

My partner at that time was spreading a fresh bale of hay and shooed Rocky away from the pile as he was shaking it out. The pony almost casually cow-kicked him in the knee, just enough to send Ken scurrying out of the pen, but not enough to have really hurt him.

"Pit Bull Pony" Strikes Again

A couple weeks after Rocky moved in, a neighbor's Rottweiler got loose—a dog that had been banned in the next county for running cows. I was too far away when it happened to do anything, and I watched in horror as the dog crouched and approached the pony from behind. Even though I was yelling, running toward them, Rocky remained motionless. Suddenly, the dog leaped at his flank. I immediately imagined the worst, but Rocky got his hind legs up and under that dog, sending him flying almost to the fence line, like some sort of Bruce Lee move. And before the dog even hit the ground, Rocky had spun and was charging at him, mouth wide open with some sort of "horse-growl" coming out of him that I have never heard, before or after. To be honest, I was now scared for the dog; I was still yelling—but now at Rocky. I was sure he was going to end that Rottweiler's life. The horse caught my eye for a split second…and something happened. He paused ever so little in his charge and that second gave the dog his only chance to escape. (We never saw the dog on our property again.)

Rocky approached the fence then, still looking at me. I think that was the first time I truly "saw" him for who he was. I realized this horse was not like any other.

He reached across the fence to where I stood, awe-struck and unsure. I had my hand in a "fist-bump" position—a safety precaution inspired by his recent biting episode with my daughter. He touched his muzzle to my knuckles in one, definite and clear moment, then looked into my eyes again. Blowing out a big breath, he turned and looked back over his shoulder at Dakota, who stood apart, away from all the action that had just taken place, then back at me. I felt a jolt of warmth go through my body.

Honestly, I teared up.

Unceremoniously, in what I would eventually come to understand as Rocky's way to "end the lesson," he sauntered off. I felt at that moment I had experienced something truly amazing, but I had no idea what it was. All I knew was that nothing this little horse did was anything other than 100 percent deliberate.

How on Earth?

When I first met Rocky, I was at the point in my career as a riding instructor, rehabilitation supervisor, EAL teacher, and clinician where I thought I had a good handle on all things horse.

But I was on the Bunny Slope and Rocky was about to take me on the Black Diamond Trail. Up until then, I had worked on figuring out kinder and gentler ways to work with horses. I had a lot of tools in my tool belt to get a horse "on board." But I was about to come to understand that I was still just getting horses to do what I wanted in nice ways *but not really hearing them*. I had years of conditioning that told me to think, "Horse, now that I showed up, *my* agenda is the only game in town."

At the same time, the majority theory at the moment agreed that humans must be the dominant role, no matter what. For safety's sake, the horse needs to know that he can't "get away with it," whatever "it" is, ever.

My brain kept asking, "How on Earth can you truly have an *authentic* relationship with this dominance mentality?" It also asked, "How on Earth can you have a *safe* relationship without relying on dominance?"

This was like the picture of the snake eating his own tail.

Tell It Like It is

What Rocky did was demonstrate amazing self-control. He was not above telling me exactly what he thought.

Yet, all the things people want to do with a horse generally rely upon the horse *doing* them. For instance, taking Rocky out for a walk was fine until he wanted grass. I had plenty of "skating" incidents as Rocky took me to where the grass was greenest. Then, when he was done, he would walk me home.

You could ride Rocky…if Amber and Dakota were going out for a trail ride with you. Otherwise, he didn't really see the point.

At no point was there any sense of ill will; Rocky never completely got angry about anything. Yet, he never really let me touch him. There was a distance that I had never experienced before with a horse. I was really "missing it," whatever "it" was. He was a tough read.

To Do or Not to Do

He looked like a teddy bear as winter approached. His coat had two layers to it. He got fuzzy like a woolly mammoth. This made me wish he was happier with me, and friendlier, because I just wanted to love on him.

As the weeks I had Rocky became a year, and the year dragged on, I went through every tool in my tool belt. Clicker training got his attention, but it made him muggy and demanding. Nothing I did made him interested in "pleasing" me. He had no vested interest in my praise on any level. Therefore, any training methods that used pressure to make "the wrong thing hard and the right thing easy" simply didn't work, because he never agreed that the right thing was now easy. (The right thing was still hard because he didn't want to do it.)

He learned what I expected of him, and conformed to a degree, but I could not reach the soul of this horse.

One day, we had a great deal of snow fall quickly over an hour or two. Rocky's hay was totally covered, and I looked out the window to see he was using his hoof to clear it away. I went outside with a shovel to help him, and as he watched me clear his food pile, he did something different: He blew out his nose and flopped his ears to the side. I just "knew" deep within me that this was Rocky's version of saying some version of, "Thank you."

Before I went back to the house, Rocky left the hay and followed me a little way. I had learned that he seemed to like to have his ears rubbed, so I offered that. He hung around for a bit, then did his usual unceremonious turn away and went back to his hay.

I thought about what had happened long and hard. It occurred to me: I was interested in what *he* was interested in—namely his hay. He showed me connection when I showed him I cared about what *he* cared about.

Hmm…

All the time I had been with this horse, I had been trying to get him to care about what *I* cared about. If I went to him with an agenda, that meant he could not do the things he liked or that were important to him. He liked to do things on *his* terms, but anything I wanted to do with him was on *my* terms. I had been thinking of him as a "stubborn" pony, but now a light dawned on me: Eating hay was *his* thing, yet I never stuck around and shared in that with him. What if I started to make time to just *be present* with Rocky, observing what he thought was important? I began to watch him differently. I lingered more often and tried to pay attention to whatever it might be that *he* was paying attention to.

One day I started a round-pen session to give Rocky a little exercise, when suddenly, I noticed he kept turning to look at me. The "look" had the air of a question to it. Stopping the session, I wondered what was wrong—what was he looking at? I approached him to offer a rub and a stroke, and he leaned away from me, then stepped off to the side. I thought maybe he wanted to run a little and stepped back to send him off—but he gave me that look again! After a few more attempts, I finally realized that he was showing me some-thing that was important to him: his personal space.

Feeling overwhelmed and like I probably had no right training horses, I sat down on a dry spot in the round pen. Rocky wasted no time in approaching me, but as soon as I felt a little overwhelmed by his approach—I must have flinched—he stopped at that exact moment. The light bulb was flickering in my brain. Was this what *he* felt like when I approached *him*?

AHA MOMENT

There is a saying in the school of Zen that a student must be open to Zen "like an uncarved block." This means you agree to know nothing. It is a state of pure potential.

With Rocky, I decided to agree to know nothing. I was starting anew.

One day, I was sitting in the paddock with Rocky as he ate his hay (I was now committed to spending quality time with him, doing things *he* liked), when he left the pile he was munching to wander over and see what I was doing.

What I was doing—besides sitting near him and appreciating hay-eating—was reading a book about horses, in yet another attempt to find some sort of elusive nugget of insight. Rocky looked right into my eyes, a curious expression on his face. How do you explain reading to a horse? I told him out loud, "Reading is like eating for your mind."

Rocky actually bit the book at that moment, pulling it out of my hands. I smiled up at him as he made a grimacing face. It didn't appear to taste good. And right then and there I experienced one of those crystal-clear moments, when you just "know" what your horse is thinking. He was saying to me, "If you really want to know horses, you should ask a horse."

Of course! How ridiculous it is to ask *people* to explain *horses*! There was one problem, though: How exactly did you "ask a horse"?

Rocky positioned himself over my shoulder as I remained seated in my lawn chair. Hanging his lovely head over me, he closed his eyes and started to breathe very deeply. I began to copy him: eyes closed, breathing deeply, feeling my rib cage expanding. It seemed like my lower ribs got larger and fuller somehow. The sensation was wonderful, and I smiled and opened my eyes, reaching out to pat him. He put his ears back, and nudged my hand away, looking cross.

Okay—I got it. I went back to deep breathing. After a few minutes I again came out of my meditative state and tried to connect with him. Again, he corrected me. This happened several times until I finally realized that the deep breathing *was* the connection.

So I settled into my first taste of Zero.

Standing up, I moved toward him, but stopped as soon as he flinched. I stepped backward—and he approached me...and stopped when *I* flinched.

Wow!

I was teaching classes at a horse rescue that weekend, and I brought this newfound awareness into a pen with a horse that was impossible to catch. After skating around the edge of his "bubble of personal space" for about 10 minutes, listening to him like I had started to listen to Rocky, he walked right over to me.

Double wow!

That started a whole cascade of epiphanies.

Starting Over

Once Rocky had introduced me to Zero, I started looking for it everywhere. I now realized why he was so often "not into" what I wanted to do with him: I was incredibly tense in my body language. I had no idea I was physically tense because I didn't feel tense emotionally. Working with Rocky, I learned to round my shoulders ("O" posture) and breathe into my floating ribs when I was near him. When I did this, he hung around, went for a ride, did what I wanted. If I didn't, he got difficult.

As *he* trained *me*, he was making the wrong thing hard and the right thing easy!

I began to watch him closely for other "signals" that I could copy. One day I noticed that when I approached, he would wiggle his lips. I saw him lip wiggling at Dakota and at my cat and even sometimes when he was standing all by himself in the sunshine. So, I decided to wiggle my lips, too.

I approached his paddock, paused, made an "O" posture, and wiggled away. Rocky's ears perked right up, and for the first time *ever*, he *trotted over to the gate*!

What had just happened? He had rewarded me for learning, and I started using the lip wiggle all over the place. Over time and many uses, I figured out that it meant, "I am having a nice day. Want to share it with me?"

So I began to use lip wiggling in all my other work with horses, as well as Zero and the "O" posture. My students and clients were willing to try out my new "wild" ideas, and they, too, began to see results.

Rocky Road

My next step in learning from Rocky was to only ride him bareback. I knew I was learning so much about his body language and my body language that it felt like the saddle was in the way. At the same time, I decided to go bitless because I was starting to believe that if I couldn't use body language to communicate with my horse, I had no business hiding behind tools like bits.

Rocky seemed to love the idea of me being "all natural" on him—especially because he could snatch leaves and grass without me being able to do anything about it! I couldn't keep my Zero when he was gorging himself. I knew I had to figure out a way for us to come to an agreement about this. This was a true horsemanship challenge: I didn't want to resort to pure dominance and go all the way back to a "my way or the highway" mentality, but I also didn't want him taking over as he was now. We had to reach a middle ground.

Where was the beginning place for us to really talk to each other while I was riding him? I decided to model a starting place after the first lesson Rocky had taught me: I got on and then just sat there, breathing deeply, expanding my floating ribs, and finding Zero. Rocky stood with me for a few minutes; then he had his own idea. He walked a small circle, came back to the mounting block, and stopped there. I knew he was saying, "Get off."

So, I got off. Frustrated, I threw my arms up in the air and asked out loud, "What? What do you want?"

Rocky blew out his nose, then touched the ground with his muzzle, gently bobbing his head.

In round-pen situations, I had frequently seen horses giving this same signal before approaching me. I had also seen Rocky do it when he was with Dakota if she got jumpy. Not knowing what else to do, I bent over next to him, touching the ground with my fingers. Rocky lingered there, sniffing my fingers and then the back of my head, which was lowered next to his. Then he lifted his head, licking his lips. So I did, too.

Honestly, sometimes it felt like he was Anne Sullivan and I was Helen Keller.

Rocky blew out his nose, flopped his ears to the side, and looked at the mounting block. I got on it, but before I could mount, he moved away. I got off the block, and he came back to it. I stepped on it, and waited. He waited, too. Then I noticed he was lightly stepping from side to side with his front feet. I stepped side to side, too, swaying a little. I made more of an "O" posture and breathed out. Rocky dropped his head to the ground and let out a loud snort. Then he moved *into* my leg, pressing his body against it.

His whole body changed, seeming to get warmer and friendlier. I felt "invited."

Slowly swinging up and sitting on his back, I used my "O" posture to stay soft and relaxed. He breathed up into me, lifting my body slightly with every breath. It was an amazing feeling. Then I picked up the reins. He put his ears back and tightened up.

Whoops!

I got off and went back to the side-to-side sway on the mounting block. Again, he invited me onto his back. Now I wondered if something about the way I was holding the reins was not right. I had grown up riding English, and in my dressage lessons I had learned to use the four reins of the double bridle. I also had ridden enough Western to be comfortable with a nice "float" in the reins. I didn't think my hands were hard or demanding. I really didn't know what could be wrong.

Slowly, I lifted the reins from where they hung on Rocky's withers. I tried making more of an "O" posture with my upper body, my palms facing a little more downward so that my thumbs almost touched. Instantly, he lowered his head, relaxing his neck and shoulders. I returned my hands to their "normal" position (thumbs on top) and Rocky tensed up. Even with loose reins and no bit, he commented about the posture I used—there was something about the upright thumbs that he disagreed with.

Now, on the surface, this flew in the face of about every riding school out there. However, after that session with Rocky I reviewed hundreds of images of advanced riders from every school of thought, both old and new. I looked at historic pictures from the 1920s, 30s, and 40s, as well as ancient illustrations of baroque riders from all over Europe. I included as many disciplines as I could find: classical dressage, bullfighting, cutting, and reining. I looked at every-thing—good, bad, and ugly—to try to broaden my base of reference. I looked at the riders' hands and arms and how they related to the "shape" of their horses: some horses lifted their necks from the base, some were overbent, some were low-headed, while others didn't seem collected at all.

In my research, I tried to focus on the horse-and-rider pairs that looked "together." In these instances I would often also find a slight variation in posture: a turn of the hands or softening of the arms into what I now recognized as an "O" while riding. When the rider's palms faced *slightly* downward, they allowed the shoulder blades to open, the rider's breath to deepen, and the rider's lower body to "connect" to the upper body. I realized that this was how the rider could "sink" the core downward and make his back firm. Even in still pictures, I could see the core energy of these riders tucked in and down. It was not contracted and stiff at all but "alive" and absorbing the energy of the horse.

I could now see that some other riders looked like two halves—upper and lower—and their horses looked disconnected from back to front.

All over the world and within any number of different riding traditions, this natural effect happened. Yet, no one talked about it.

Tai Chi Strikes Again

In Tai Chi, the fountain of power comes out of the *Tantien* or *Hara*—the core. Tai Chi focuses on an "O"-type posture for power that is soft and causes the human to fill with positive *chi* (good energy). You are taught to sink your core in and downward, with your arms and legs becoming extensions of it. In beginner Tai Chi, you often learn to "hold the ball," in which you "embrace" a big, imaginary, beach ball and move around a room with your arms held that way. You then connect your movements down to your feet, so that your whole body is communicating clearly, and your core is the conductor of the orchestra.

As an experiment, I tried going through my Tai Chi forms holding my thumbs up as I had been taught to do in riding position. It didn't work at all. In fact, it made the lower half of my body uncoordinated.

So, as riders, why were we taught to hold our bodies in the ways we have? I realized I had to go past the idea of "correct" position on horseback and look at riding from the point of view of *body language*, not showmanship.

From the perspective of body language, when we hold our hands out with the thumbs up and our elbows in, our hard-wired response is to limit our breathing and utilize our biceps. We are in a classic push-pull posture. The subtlety of the muscle arrangements in our bodies and the naturally "automated" responses that our bodies have are amazing. I picked the brains of physical therapists and chiropractors, body builders and yoga instructors, asking for their insight regarding the human body's ability to maneuver. I learned that when you stabilize your upper body to the point of immobility, you could still move your lower half. This allowed us to carry items while walking great distances, as we would have needed as a nomadic species in the past. However, when the upper body begins to move around, the lower half *must* move to compensate for balance. In other words, by loosening up your arms and hands, your core and legs *must* adapt and rebalance. Otherwise, you would fall over.

This helped make sense of the "O" posture Rocky seemed to want me to practice. If the posture was detectable in skilled riders who looked "like one" with their horses, then I felt there must be a "body wisdom" principle behind it—something related to the subconscious, innate controls that prevent us from falling over. I wanted to link my conscious mind to my subconscious responses so I could engage this body wisdom fully and be completely present for my horse's body. I wanted my natural ability to balance to add value to my horse's desire to stay balanced. While I didn't *feel* like I was stiff and I'd always prided myself on having a light feel on the reins, my body language had transmitted a signal to Rocky that he didn't care for. However, simply rotating my hands slightly allowed a softness to travel from my core up my arms to my shoulders and clavicle, and this then automatically softened my breathing. When riding him, I began to feel as though Rocky and I were flowing forward together quite naturally.

I realized Rocky was teaching me about riding a horse, not how to perform a specific discipline. He was spelling out how to connect with my own body wisdom, and I decided I would follow the advice of a horse, instead of the advice of people *about* horses. Since I am not in the military and I am not an active competitor, I am free to ride a horse as befits me, but training and tradition was pretty ingrained, and I struggled a bit. I decided to bring elements of this discovery to some of my students to test it out.

But Does It Work?

When I introduced the "O" and slightly altered hand position in the saddle to my students, I was floored by the results. First, the effect on the horses was dramatic and immediate. I had my students rotate their hands until their palms faced completely downward, and instructed them to "hold" the Tai Chi ball (giving them the "O" posture) as they moved around the arena. The changes appeared to ground them. The horses immediately released stress by breathing more deeply, reaching out with the head, neck, and shoulders, and taking even, relaxed steps. They became so relaxed that some of them yawned.

When I asked my students what they were feeling, everyone agreed that they felt much less tense, or that they had not realized how tense they must usually be. Now their deep breathing could circulate much more effectively. While at first I told the riders to go ahead and allow their bodies to relax into a little slump if it helped create the "O," most very quickly found a new relationship with their backs. This posture did not sacrifice their backs; in fact, they found they could easily use their core to create a straight, flat back because their upper body was so soft.

Next, I worked to understand how to keep this newfound openness through a turn. The common adaptation people often use of drawing the hand across the thigh for a tighter turn completely unbalances the horse. Drawing the hand and arm backward activates the bicep, creating tightness, and drawing it across your thigh sends a message down the inside front leg of the horse in a way that limits that leg's movement. However, keeping the palm facing down and drawing the hand out and away from the Mid-Neck Button (see p. 42) at the height of your own core not only balances the horse's front end, it initiates the same natural arc the horse would move on when on his own. In other words, when a horse is naturally changing directions when loose, he uses his head and neck like a ballast, bending around from the Mid-Neck Button. If the rider copies this motion, he can create tremendous liberty in the forehand. In addition, once we reconnected the dots to the use of leg cues, I found the students' bodies were already working with the turn, and their legs were already using the correct set of balancing aids. The phenomena of innate body wisdom added tremendous value to the conscious use of leg aids.

Of course, my students could not ride in a horse show like this, so I needed to work on their muscle memory—the horse needed their body language to feel a certain way, with a sense of openness, even when they had adopted a more traditional position for competition.

After a few weeks of practicing, we refined the motions down to a more classical look. However, the slight shift of awareness was still in all of our bodies and hands, and the horses felt it. The gentle rotation of the hands toward a palms-down position was "invisible," and we were ready for the intercollegiate show.

To the Show!

When it comes to intercollegiate competition, shows are run by groups of colleges who each take turns hosting. At each event, there are a limited number of horses for the day, and everyone rides them. Competitors are assigned a horse but are not allowed to touch or meet him until it is their turn. By the end of the day, the horses are spent, tired of the revolving door of riders, and can get quite edgy.

While some colleges were considered "horsey" schools with scouted talent on their teams, ours was not one of them. Frequently our riders had only just learned to ride in the previous semester. There were also some students who had an extensive background in riding and horsemanship, which meant I needed to address the needs of both highly talented riders and brand-new ones. I also wanted all my students to have fun and come out of the ring after their ride believing that for those seven minutes, they gave something lovely back to the horse.

Above all, I wanted everyone to stay safe. It was not uncommon for a tired and bored horse to buck toward the end of the day.

One of my least experienced students was given a horse that had bucked in the previous session. She was nervous; she considered sitting her round out. At the last minute, her gumption drove her to try, and she mounted up. On the way to the gate, I watched as she turned her palms so they faced totally downward and took several deep breaths in an "O," lightly turning the horse's head from side to side to release the tension in his poll. At the gate, she reverted to the "correct" position and in they went. The horse cruised around the arena as though the two had been together all along. He was not a pretty mover, but his ears were in a contented sideways position as my student continued to focus on all her calm-down cues. She was only in the walk-trot division, having had only one semester of riding, but she came in third. The whole team was so happy for her, and I was sold on the process. If nothing else, the altered upper body positions seemed to increase the level of safety for riders as it increased the level of comfort for horses.

Thank you, Rocky.

What Else?

In the hours I had spent pouring over old pictures and writings as I tried to make sense of what I was learning from little Rocky, I had contemplated another aspect of equitation, this one related to dressage and its goal of activating the horse's core and hind end. The desired effect was that the horse "sit down" in his movement, using his hind end to power forward and up and his core to lift the rider in a constant rolling sensation. This liberated the horse's front end and made the horse capable of performing airs above the ground and beautiful, ballet-like movements, such as piaffe and passage. The neck of the horse looks arched, the base of the neck has lifted in engagement so that the chest is exposed, and the shoulders are free to move.

I could see that this, the ultimate horse and rider experience, was totally at Zero. To achieve this level of power without losing control, the riders needed to become more and more still internally, and the horses were encouraged to "lend" their powerful movements to the rider without becoming aggressive. Of course, in battle, where dressage originated, aggression was useful, but not if it was out of control.

As an artist, my eye tends to pick up certain details in figures. In many of the photos and illustrations of advanced dressage work I studied, I noticed that often the wing bones (scapulae) of the riders were rotated backward and their hands and arms were curled slightly inward.

I searched through the Tai Chi moves I knew, and sure enough, I hit upon the "reverse ball" arm rotation. This sank your *Tantien* down and anchored your lower body so deeply that in a real Tai Chi master application, the master was immoveable. I realized I used the arm position mostly when trying to get as many grocery bags as I could into my arms so I only had to make one trip from the car to the house. In this "scoop" position, your humerus rotates outward, turning the "eye" of the inner elbow forward, engaging the scapula, as well as the *subscapularis* tendon (which goes up into your armpit). This, in turn, can collect the *transverse abdominis* muscle in your abdominal wall (centered on top of the pubic bone). In other words, simply rotating my arms by turning my thumbs out "told" my pelvis to engage. My legs were indeed quite anchored.

Scoop It Up

I got on Rocky and adopted the "scoop-up" position. Allowing the core of my body to follow his natural motion, I realized it wanted to tuck in and down. My lower back deepened, and my own "poll" (below my occipital bone at the base of my skull) wanted to lengthen and arc. My legs wrapped around him comfortably but with a lot of focus.

Using a Tai Chi motion called "wave hands like clouds," I emphasized one side of the "scoop" (rotating my thumb, humerus, and scapula in one, fluid motion) more than the other to see what would happen. Rocky became very supple beneath me, and I could follow the feeling from one hand diagonally through my body to the other seat bone. This sensation flowed down the opposite leg, and if I lifted my big toe a little, the anchoring of the bilateral movement my body was making seemed to complete the wave motion. I followed the feel and timing of this movement in my own body with a soft inner core that allowed Rocky to arc first one way and then the other with ease. By playing with the level of rotation in my core, or the amount of leg aid, we could bend in an arc more or less, or from the front or hind. Essentially, it felt like doing Tai Chi *with* my horse, not just *on* my horse.

When I released all cues and returned to neutral, Rocky took a few straight steps forward. And then I felt something truly amazing: It was like his whole hind end shuffled underneath me and his front end lifted in front of me. His back seemed to lift beneath me and a pleasant rolling sensation carried me forward. He began to march forward with his poll arched, moving with what felt like pride.

We rode around like that for a few more minutes, and suddenly his lower back cracked like a self-adjustment. He blew out his nose and shook his head a little. I got off and rubbed his ears. We were both quite pleased.

I went on to experiment with how the "scoop" motion might work when leading a horse, as well. While leading Rocky forward, I invited him to respond to my thumb-to-arm-to-scapula rotation (as though I was scooping out some ice cream from a big bin). What happened was interesting: He abruptly softened his neck and bent in the direction of my suggestion. Since we were walking forward, this made him soften his head and neck and bend *toward* me. In the interest of exploration, I offered the "scoop" while changing direction, and while both beginning to walk off and coming to a halt. In each case, the "scoop" created a softening effect while encouraging him to bend, yield, or comply in a relaxed manner. I did note that the effect was lost if I forgot to begin with my palm *facing down* on the lead rope (thumb toward the ground), however. Leading with my thumb in the upright position (pointing toward the halter) seemed to send an instant message to Rocky to brace, even when there was a "float" in the lead rope. I realized my own body language was unconsciously in the position of fighting or bracing when my thumb was up because my bicep was engaged. I had uncovered a secret stash of tension that I was accidentally including in all my horse-handling skills. Maybe I was not feeling *emotionally* tense, but my body was sending a different message…and Rocky was not happy with it.

Rocky was more than willing to explore both my palm-down and scoop-up motions on the ground. It seemed to help him feel less frustrated with being led. Over time, these two motions ended up smoothing out most of the tangles we tended to get into in hand.

When I rotated my wrists palm down while leading, it created a relaxing, soothing, and anchoring feel on the line. I realized this was part of my "O" posture on the ground. The "scoop" on the ground gave me a tremendous advantage if a horse was determined to run away with me (not uncommon at the rescues where I worked). I learned that by creating this "scoop" movement with a horse that was tense, afraid, or difficult, a resistance-free message went through the lead rope, causing the horse to turn back toward me rather than try to flee or fight. Eventually, I realized that using the "scoop" while facing a horse and asking him to back up could soften and relax his back and hind end, or create a very easy bend from any point on his body. The overall effect of these practices was to change leading a horse from a task into a dance.

I was pleased to discover that even previously hard-to-lead horses responded to this new approach very quickly and that students and volunteers I worked with could learn it just as fast. As opposed to training techniques that are usually based on obedience, the use of palm-down and scoop-up on the lead rope became quite natural after only a short time using it. It seemed to me that it gave such a pleasant sensation to both horses and humans so quickly that there was really nothing to learn! All you had to do was feel the ease and comfort of this body language once or twice, and then your inner body wisdom took over and you essentially couldn't remember to do it "wrong."

As I deepened my awareness of what had previously been subconscious body language while riding, certain types of riding styles began to make sense. It was like the "secret sauce" of body wisdom that was hiding underneath any discipline began to instantly pop out at me: I could understand the synthesis of body language to riding style. What I might have previously considered just a certain set of rules pertaining to a given riding system now appeared to me as logical adaptations, springing forth from the deeper level of body mechanics that made up the original body language of a master rider. Whether I watched a talented Western rider rounding up cows or a classical dressage maestro, there were—beneath the obvious surface differences—core similarities in body mechanics, which allowed the horse to use his own body in direct correspondence. By overexaggerating the motions of "O" or "X" and palm-down or scoop-up, and by keeping it very, very simple, I found that I could "reach" a wide variety of horses—those I was working with at rescues and in riding schools, as well as the array of private clients I had from all walks of life. These horses came from such diverse backgrounds, and many had "holes" in their "riding horse education." But by keeping it simple, and knowing where to start, all horses relaxed about the riding process, and some made enormous turnarounds. Even highly schooled horses took bigger breaths and let go of that edgy, tense energy that often lies just below the surface.

Rocky had shown me a way to begin having a conversation *from the back of a horse*, rather then getting up there and expecting him to be a biological motorcycle. When we, as riders, get on our horses, we assume that they should know our cues, our aids, and our style. However, the horse is often guessing at what will make us happy—consider how one rider is satisfied with a slow, ambling walk, while another wants a spirited, lively one. Each rider's unconscious body language settles into a sense of "this movement is right," and that might be different for every person. The horse is left not knowing why people are so hard to please.

When a person is convinced her seat is correct, then the "problem" usually lands on the horse—it is his fault he is not performing something correctly.

Rocky taught me that this is very unpleasant for a horse to deal with. He made me dig deeper and realize that while I was on his back, perhaps I needed to rethink my expectations from years of riding. My trained beliefs had said to him, "I don't care what you like or are interested in. I only want you to work for me. I have not asked, nor have I given you a choice. I expect you to speed up or slow down when I demand it. And it's not over till it's over."

It occurred to me that it was impossible to treat a horse like a "partner" if I was also demanding obedience. Learning to ask Rocky permission to "come aboard" was his first lesson to me. Learning how to blend with *his* body, instead of demanding he obey mine, was next. The final picture came to light when *we*, as a truly integrated unit, could Go Somewhere Together. Then I could use no more than a piece of baling twine around his neck and still hop on and have some fun. This was the point at which he learned to move an overturned muck bucket into place with his front hoof and look at me to offer me a ride.

At the same time, the other horses in my working life were all softening, opening, and becoming more engaged in the process of their own existence. My students were beginning to be able to "hear" their horses, and even though not every single day was roses and rainbows, there were fewer and fewer incidences of horses "blowing up." In fact, this became the rarity and usually pointed to something more troublesome in that horse's world.

I could feel it all coming together. What I learned from Rocky was truly a gift.

LICK AND CHEW

By being open to allowing my horse to teach and guide me, I broke through the preconceived notions and limiting beliefs I had been bumping up against in my earlier work with horses. Submitting to a new paradigm was sometimes scary and often difficult. Allowing my "working knowledge" to be suspended was the only way to experience the breakthrough that Rocky offered me. What lay on the other side of what had been an uncomfortable learning curve was worth the effort.

Chapter 6

"O" Finds "X"

Practicing "O" with Dakota took our sessions to a whole new level. She was interested in refinement. With her, I could easily influence all four feet individually, depending upon how I rotated my arm and hand, or just my core, or when I used my "O" posture or stood up tall during groundwork. It was with Dakota that I realized the opposite of "O" is "X."

Remember that "X" posture includes high, tense shoulders, tight lips, hard eyes, breath held, tense legs. But "X" also has so many nuances and variables available to it. Depending on degree and type of use, "X" can motivate, stop, or block. It can also signal a "stay" or hold. I could keep my core in an "O" to soften but combine it with just enough "X" by engaging my arms and legs and shoulders in a little bouncy upward movement. I discovered tiny "X" postures, like pointing my finger to engage more, meant that I could explore lateral movements at liberty or on the longe line. It was like learning to drive a car: How much gas, clutch, and brake did I need? And oh, yeah, what gear should I be in?

This got exciting! With a mind toward the more elaborate liberty performances that I had witnessed, I practiced many new kinds of groundwork with Dakota.

What Are Those Spots?

I continued to study as many different disciplines as I could to see what underlying elements they all had in common. My influences ran the gamut, from stock-horse training to the horsemen of the Mongolian steppe to trick training for the movies. I bought and rented and downloaded as many videos as I could, looking for the correlating features between trainers and "horse whisperers." I turned the volume down so as not to be distracted by people's words; I could just watch their bodies in time with the horses. I watched, stopped, rewound, and watched again.

I began to see that, in order to influence the horse, people used the same spots on the horse's body. They might use different methods, but they were the same spots. So why were these the "magic spots"?

Rocky had already taught me to ask horses, so I returned to the herd.

AHA MOMENT

My herd had grown as I had adopted three more horses from rescues, including a mare in foal. With this little family group, I had the opportunity to try to uncover the secrets I was looking for. The new herd members all had a difficult past, but of course the baby had no knowledge of this at all. Watching how the horses came together to teach and nurture the filly was invaluable. Rocky doted on her. In fact, he became the Mentor for the whole group. I would occasionally add other horses to the herd for a few months at a time while I was helping them and their owners, and Rocky and I would work together on finding the right ways to connect.

One day, I realized Rocky had used three of the "magic spots" in a row to first ask the filly to move off in a certain direction, and then to tell her to stop.

It was one of those lightbulb moments. These weren't "spots"—they were "Buttons." They didn't belong to any of the trainers I'd studied or to me. They belonged to the horses. The Buttons were part of *their* communication system, and we usurped them to create the training we wanted.

Quitter

As I explored the "spots" or "Buttons" on the horses, I was still thinking like a trainer. I was a kinder, gentler trainer, but I was still objectifying the horse. I was still approaching him with the attitude of, "What can I get you to do for me?"

In a moment of inspiration, I realized I had to quit. I would make my money a different way, and when it came to horses, I would dedicate myself to understanding how, why, and when they used their Buttons for their own purposes.

I stopped riding that spring and summer. I ran temporary fencing to create a path through the woods from my paddocks to a neighbor's field where I had permission to graze the horses. This allowed us to walk together through the woods to the grazing area. Often the horses would begin walking with me, then leave to gleefully gallop the trail to the field. (Walking home was usually much calmer.) I would spend two hours every day sitting and watching the herd in the field, trying to learn. I brought a camera and a sketch pad and recorded as much as I could.

However, I found that all the layers of preconceived notions reared up and became very noisy. I had to throw everything I knew and had been taught up in the air and sift through the pieces to create a brand-new pyramid of seeing, knowing, and understanding.

The Shadow of the Unknown

I had given up all my clients and did not teach or coach at the college that spring and summer. What was driving me was too strong to be ignored. I had no idea where it would lead, and had to supplement my income doing other things, but I was committed.

A few of my college students were around through the summer, and they agreed to "think-tank" with me on my project. A few times a week, they would sit in the field with me, and we would try to see what *was* there, *not* what we *thought* was there. Being college students, their minds were brimming with possibility, not already entrenched in working knowledge.

It is quite uncomfortable to be faced with the unknown. Managing six horses every day while trying to "authentically relate" with them required a certain dedication. There were still moments where I had to put halters on, or do groundwork with the filly to prepare her for human handling and the vet and farrier. Sometimes I had to "do things to" the horses, like brush the mud off or spray for bugs. But I remained as true to the idea of "non-interference" as I reasonably could otherwise.

Little by little, my team and I started to see and record more and more of how the horses used the Buttons and "X" and "O" to communicate. I was beginning to see that they had much more subtlety than I ever imagined.

I Can See Clearly Now

One day, Jag pushed into Rocky's space a little too brazenly. Jag was one of his favorite mares, but she could be pushy. He reacted a bit strongly, biting her Mid-Neck Button. It was not a bad bite, but she scooted away to the far corner and sulked over a different hay pile. After about five minutes, Rocky's whole posture changed, and he blew out his nose a few times, flopped his ears sideways and seemed to droop his shoulders—all while eating his hay. He then turned to look toward her. Her ears immediately perked up; she lifted her head, blew out her nose, too, and then touched the ground lightly with her muzzle. Her whole affect made me think if she could talk she'd be saying, "Aw shucks, can I come back now?"

Rocky lifted his head a little, and then touched the ground lightly with *his* muzzle. Jag sauntered back over to him, stopping a few feet away to look to the side and then touch the ground again, before rejoining him at his hay pile. They then touched noses very distinctly not just once, but three times. One of my students was with me that day, and after we witnessed the interaction, she and I broke into a huge dialogue about what it all meant.

As an experiment, I began to put out one, fair-sized pile of hay for a group of horses, rather than breaking it into smaller, separate piles. Repeatedly, I witnessed the pecking order and how small disagreements would get worked out, and what seemed to be "apologies" offered. Almost all the communication between the horses revolved around the few Buttons on the head and neck. There was also significance in the timing of lifting and lowering the head, how and when the horse looked away, and when the greeting touch of the muzzle was used.

I started to see that horses seemed to have a circle of communication that had a beginning, end, and renewal. There were patterns to be repeated to show connection, hierarchy, and togetherness. Each of these patterns followed a protocol, whether it was enacted over a pile of hay or while roaming around the field. Horses could start a conversation and end one. They could also pick up where they left off. I witnessed Rocky on several occasions "talking" to one mare about something, only to veer off to "talk" to another mare, then come back to the first and pick up the thread exactly where he'd left it.

While the horses were not in any hurry to communicate, it also appeared they were part of some kind of dialogue most of the time, even when standing totally still.

Now What?

I had to get into the herd and emulate their movements. I felt comfortable using "X" and "O," and I had now coined the term "Aw-Shucks" to represent a request related to pressure. It could mean, "Can you take the pressure off?" or "I will take the pressure off of you," or "I like the way you took the pressure off," or "I want you to relax more," or "I need to relax more." This movement was a comment on the level of intensity in a relationship or in a horse's relationship to the world at that moment. Of course, we are not designed to bend down and stick our noses in the dirt all day long. My close-enough equivalent was to casually dig my toe into the ground while slouching in an exaggerated "O."

When I did this posture, the horses always acknowledged it. Sometimes they came to me very softly and directly. Sometimes they dropped their muzzles to the ground. If I did it in response to a tense moment, then they might touch the dirt and blow their noses as they tried to release tension. If I was too much "X" for whatever reason, they would turn their heads slightly away and sniff the dirt. When a horse was on a lead rope and he sniffed the ground, and then my shoe, it was often followed by the horse lifting his head halfway and beginning to lean as if to move off. I came to understand this was a suggestion we go somewhere. Once I started to "hear" that request, I looked for nuances in the way a horse sniffed my boot or the angle of the head and neck—sometimes I found it was just a request for me to reposition myself. Then I had to see where the horse wanted to reposition me, which he might do by "popping" his shoulder toward me and gently lining it up to my shoulder. The next time he sniffed the ground, then my shoe, and leaned his shoulder toward me, I moved back to his shoulder all by myself…and was met with much nose-blowing and a good shake of the head and neck with a lick and chew.

I was being complimented on learning a new lesson!

Rinse and Repeat

I gradually expanded my repertoire of Horse Speak in this way. I started with a certain movement that either the horse or I initiated, and I then sought to repeat the encounter again and again and in different settings and for different reasons. Always staying open to the possibility that the horse may have reasons that I couldn't understand yet, I did my best to experience enough repetition under enough variables to confirm an essence of the meaning of that exact movement or signal. It all began to seem to make sense as I gave the movements catchy names that were easy to remember, and then located them in relation to the horse, according to the Buttons. I paid special attention to getting a handle on the protocols of each category of communication I had identified: greeting, hierarchy, bonding, movement, and ending.

In correlating what I was doing with the horses to learning a foreign language (I had taken a few years of Spanish), I could think of specific words (nouns, verbs, adjectives) but then there was grammar, tenses, and other nuances to consider. There is a formality to learning not just the words of a language, but how the language fits together to become expressive. And finally, of course, there is the art of speaking it—fluency.

Yet, under it all, I reminded myself that most of our unconscious communication—meaning that of humans—is truly through body language. If anyone has traveled and stayed in a foreign country, this becomes obvious when we revert to pointing at our mouth to ask where to get some food. This is overtly relatable by any human being. While the subtle body language of a land or culture is largely influenced by customs and traditions, you can still always wrap your arms around your body and pretend to shiver to say you are cold, and people will get it.

I was reaching for the *broadest* meanings with horses—the most obvious body language signals, like pointing to your mouth when you're hungry. How could I emulate them well enough that the horses understood me?

The funny thing was, once I got started, the horses got very chatty…

From Practice to Action

I received a phone call from the director of a local horse rescue. They had a Mustang no one could do anything with. She knew I was taking time off but asked if I could just come take a look and maybe offer some advice.

I hadn't worked with any horses outside my own herd for several months at this point. But the request didn't feel like an intrusion. Perhaps I was ready to re-enter the bigger picture.

Sure, I thought. Why not?

The little Mustang stood stoically at the back of his pen, which was attached to the barn and gave him entry to his own stall. He had buddies in pens and stalls on either side of him, but they were all separated due to specific injuries and frailties, and for the time being, needed to stay that way.

The little guy took one look at me and turned his butt toward me, dramatically and as a warning. I got it loud and clear.

Well, I thought. Here goes nothing!

I started to walk back and forth about 10 feet away from his pen, showing him all sides of me. Then I stopped and did an "Aw-Shucks."

The Mustang turned around and dropped his nose to the dirt in about two seconds!

At the time, I wasn't totally sure about the protocols yet, so I just stood there, licking and chewing with my mouth and lips. He reached his nose in the air toward me and sniffed three huffing breaths. I copied him, figuring he knew better than I did what came next. He then dramatically turned his head to the side, and so did I. Sniffing at me again, the Mustang again lowered his head, muzzle to the ground. I took it as an invitation to come over.

I scuffed my way to him in a very "O" position, and extended my arm with my hand in a fist and my knuckles up when I got close. (This "fist bump" was what I had been using in lieu of a nose to greet my horses.) He touched them lightly with his nose, and turned away, walking into his stall. The conversation seemed to be over.

I walked away to visit some of the other horses and came back a few minutes later. The Mustang was waiting for me at the fence, and he reached to touch my knuckles again. I had the old urge to pat his forehead, but this caused him to pin his ears and turn away. Oops. I hastily backed up and scuffed the ground with my toe. He responded by sniffing the ground again. Then he began to walk slowly to the left, so I did too. I stopped when he stopped, and he seemed pleased. I was curious to see what would happen if I turned to the right, so I took a step. The little horse paused a good, long moment and then swung around, also moving to the right. I didn't know what to do next, so I exhaled loudly. He started to yawn. It felt like time to take a nap, so I sat down in the dirt outside his pen. He cocked a hind leg and closed his eyes.

What would Rocky do now? I wondered. I thought of Rocky flopping his ears sideways and wiggling his lips. I couldn't flop my ears, but I could wiggle my lips, so I did. The Mustang came out of his reverie and then flopped his ears and wiggled his lips, too. This caused another round of yawning. I took a deep breath, opening my floating ribs to allow in more air, and his lower belly took a Shuddering Breath and expanded, making him look fatter for a minute.

Not sure of what else to do, I stood up. He seemed to know I was at a loss, so he swished his tail at me and headed back inside his stall. I swished my hand down by my thigh in response, and he paused, looking over his shoulder at me, and swished his tail again while blowing out his nose.

I wasn't sure what good this did the little Mustang, but I was over the moon! The volunteers who had been watching were full of questions, so I agreed to come back for a teaching day to go over some of the movements I had used and why.

I got another call the very next day: The Mustang had met a volunteer at the door of his stall in the morning, for the first time since he had arrived. He allowed a handler to place his halter on so he could go out to the bigger field. The rescue director said he was much more relaxed—it seemed like he just suddenly "fit in."

I was thrilled—but surprised. How could one visit in which I hadn't even touched him have caused such a change? Was I just lucky, or was this really happening?

Yeah, but Try to Teach It

I presented a series of mini clinics at the rescue, using the knowledge I had accrued to help the rehabilitators build rapport with the animals in their care. This made me streamline the "horse language" data I had taken in and helped me figure out how to offer it to people in a sequence that was learnable. I now knew that horses begin and end different dialogues all day long, but for the purpose of coming to an understanding with a horse, where should we begin and how?

Any one conversation with a horse could take up to 20 minutes to complete, or conversely, be over in 30 seconds! Horses say things quickly or slowly as suits them. However, the wide range of speed and levels of intensity they may use means the pattern gets lost to us. (There is risk in even using the word "pattern" here because as human beings, it encourages us to want to use it. Patterns are like blueprints, and they serve to get us to a goal. I am always trying to find ways to describe Horse Speak so that it removes the temptation to usurp. "Protocol" implies more consciousness than "pattern.") What I have come to witness is that horses use their own system in a very conscious way, and by following their protocols, I have been delighted to discover that most horses begin to relate to me completely differently within a few moments.

I had to come up with a way to enter conversations with horses that was predictable, repeatable, and that let the horses know we humans were attempting to talk to them—albeit with a thick accent. Then it hit me: We were now attempting to *talk*, not just get what we wanted, or make something happen. The little Mustang had showed me that day I spent with him *exactly* where we should begin: by saying "Hello," of course!

But how do I teach people to say "Hello" to a horse when I have seen it take 20 minutes or 30 seconds, and when I have seen horses do three or more sequences in order to say one thing? It felt overwhelming. But the horses at the rescues seemed to thrive on the few protocols I did understand. It seemed that as soon as I or the other volunteers even attempted to "talk," the horses at the rescue felt safer and more willing to do what we asked.

For the Second Act

I returned to the college to teach and coach, and picked up a few Equine Assisted Learning classes for younger students at a local therapeutic riding center, as well. This was my chance to really bring my new work to the table in terms of building rapport between horses and humans. My goal was to not only make the session good for my students but also to engage the horses in such a way as to allow them to bring their natural empathy to the lesson. Horses communicate with their bodies, but the essence of what they must talk about implies feelings. They *feel* the world around them, and they respond to life based on how they feel. They are feeling creatures.

Whenever big ideas turn into systems of learning, you lose some of the art of it, but you gain a perspective that others can follow. The service Horse Speak can provide is worth it. I never wanted to keep it all to myself; I only hope that this is just the tip of the iceberg. There are surely more and more layers to be discovered and enjoyed as time goes by.

AHA MOMENT

By using what I was now calling Horse Speak, I could ensure that horses were comfortable with my level in the pecking order (and would follow my lead in all decisions), *and* that they were emotionally available to offer empathy.

I realized from teaching students with learning disabilities that some brains interpret body language better than others. That was the big secret. Talented "horse whisperers" could decode and encode horse body language very quickly. If I could quantify the decoding and encoding process as a system, it would be teachable and learnable, instead of mystical.

Sunlight

Rocky still lives with me and his group of mares and one gelding. Sometimes, when I am finally home from teaching or a trip to some distant barn or conference, I can take a deep breath. My feet find their way out to his world, and I sniff his neck. He usually sniffs me back, sometimes gently licking the back of my hand. Dakota elegantly steps up and asks me to play with her, and the others mill around, like a school of fish, forming a tighter and tighter circle, until I am surrounded. They begin to groom each other, reaching right over me, as I apply my hands to whatever itchy spot is closest. They move carefully with me in the center of their world, taking turns to allow me to reach and touch each of them.

Sometimes, at the end of the day, just as the sun is setting, Rocky and I escape into the woods together. I have a halter and set of clip-on reins, but they just rest across his withers as we move off onto the well-worn trail. We may go far, or only a short distance, but it doesn't matter, because we choose how we spend each moment *together*.

I can still be awed by a flawless jumping round or Grand Prix freestyle to the right music. And liberty performances with multiple horses leaping and dancing are certainly inspirational to watch. But these days the sunlit treetops and quiet ambling with my best friend are all I seek. The trust and bond that we have built together is beyond any trick I could ever learn or teach. And besides, his immense wisdom is not done with me...yet.

LICK AND CHEW

I wanted to demystify the world of "horse whispering." Although it could be inspirational and beautiful, simply relying on "intuition" to work with horses left a lot of people wondering what to do next. It was often implied that some "guru" had the right magic, and if we were *lucky*, some of that magic might rub off on us.

I had begun to crack the code of Horse Speak, and what it promised was that anyone could learn to approximate equine language. It wasn't about whispering anymore. It was about having conversations.

Chapter 7

The Truth Is Out There

Puppy Pile

We all know horses are not dogs. Many of us wish they were. You've surely seen a "puppy pile" at some point, but have you ever seen a pile of foals? The inherent difference between dogs and horses is that dogs get right into each other's and our space, usually in the most pleasing of ways. Horses do not do this amongst themselves, so when a horse is acting like a puppy, he has adopted the behavior as an adaptation to accidental mixed messages people are often sending. Horses have no idea how to crawl into your lap like a dog and so a little space invasion can cause a lot of harm.

An upbeat, warm-hearted man had trailered a horse to my clinic. He had a Mustang and had worked diligently with this horse for a few years. This man—I'll call him Dave—had a very respected trainer that he brought the horse to from time to time to get "tune-ups."

Within a month or so after a tune-up, however, many of this horse's "problems" would start to re-emerge.

The Mustang, who I'll call Timmy, lived with an older mare that normally kept him calm. Without this mare with him at the clinic, Timmy found it hard to settle down.

I watched Dave's cheery face as he chuckled uncomfortably, shaking his head and mumbling, "There goes my Timmy…. He just does that!"

I asked Dave how much round penning he did with his horse, and he replied that although he would get Timmy to move out in the pen at the beginning of time they spent together, his instructions from his trainer were to only ask for a few changes of direction and a couple of trot and canter circles. He explained that if he didn't "get Timmy's bucks out," the horse was often nippy and too uptight to ride. He wouldn't even bother to ride Timmy some days because it seemed like he would never settle down.

Dave told me that his trainer was careful to keep Dave calm and had him practice deep breathing when they worked together. Dave was sure that he was following these instructions, and so he was simply baffled that Timmy was still, after so many years, acting out in this way.

On the surface, this heartbreaking situation would seem to most people to be truly the case of an unruly horse that was "just that way." Dave obviously adored his horse, and the trainer they went to was well-known for his thoughtful approach to horsemanship. No one was beating the Mustang, or rushing him, or trying to scare him into submission. It sounded like even the mare that lived with him back home was very patient and kind.

I needed to use the Greeting Ritual to see if I could diagnose what Timmy's issues really were.

The Barn Is on Fire

At my clinics, I always begin by talking about a few things before we get started. When everyone is packed into a small space together, sitting in chairs, I will often comment that although people may be seated close together, no one is touching. Even married couples and best friends are not sitting on each other's laps. As a species, we are keenly aware of our personal space, and so are horses. If dogs access the side of our nature that likes closeness, then horses access the side of our nature that needs security through personal space.

Furthermore, not only do horses and humans need personal space defined and respected, we also both need the environment we are in to be secure.

If the barn suddenly caught fire during a clinic, we would not be continuing to have a conversation. Instead, everyone would scramble to get out, possibly even knocking each other over. When horses scramble to escape what they deem a dangerous situation, they try to avoid knocking each other down. To make sure they can do this whenever and wherever they need, preserving the herd, horses practice navigating each other's personal space all day long.

The need for the environment to be secure is so strong in horses that if nothing is done to prove their world is safe, most of them will remain skeptical of their surroundings.

Remember what we learned in chapter 2: Humans walk into a new barn and instantly identify all the objects in the space—doors, brushes, floor mats, halters, lead ropes, electrical cords. We name all the things, claiming "ownership" over anything in our environment, thus deeming them non-threatening since we know what they are. Horses do not objectify the world in this way. They express ownership over objects once they have inspected them (by feeling free to touch or manipulate the object) but they do not generalize objects for the most part or until they have had enough experience with similar objects to warrant generalized learning. In other words, one horse trailer is not *any* horse trailer. One brush is not *any* brush.

Horses have a direct experience of the world, so their thoughts are more likely to flow out: "This wiggly thing [lead rope] smells like me and my person…this is mine…." Or, "The water in this bucket tastes *good*. Water in that bucket does not smell the same. It is a pleasure drinking good water."

Horses cannot have a direct relationship with us until they have confirmed that their immediate environment is safe. If they are led in and out of a barn every day for a year but never get to explore the environment and touch any items in the area, they will never be entirely certain those items are safe.

Before she told him to go ahead and run, a horse's mother would have touched everything as she inspected a new pasture with her tiny baby at her side. If you turn a horse loose in a new pen or paddock, he will usually walk around and sniff and inspect each post, rock, and tree before he has decided the area is safe. This behavior is so predictable, in fact, that simply copying it is the surest way to tell a horse that you—like his mother—have inspected the area and determined all is well.

If the barn is on fire in the horse's mind, it is going to be tough to say hello. Simply ignoring a horse for a few minutes while he is in his stall and banging around outside, inspecting the items in the aisle and hanging from the doors, is the fastest way to impress him. If you act like you own the place, he will find you very interesting, and you will have the upper hand in convincing him you are a benevolent leader who is looking out for any bogeyman that might want to harass him. While escorting a horse into a new environment, you can take the time to lead him around and let him see and smell posts, signs or racks on the wall, buckets, trunks, and so on. As you kick and manipulate the objects with a determined demeanor, your horse will watch you closely to see what else you "own." If you invite him to "own" those things, too, he will begin to "buddy up" with you (seeing as you have such power over these objects!).

I know several people who now bring their horses on walks around showgrounds early, just to give them time to literally "kick some posts" in front of their horses while no one is looking! They all agree their horses are much calmer during competition when they do this.

Timmy's Round Pen Is on Fire

This is where I began with our friend Timmy the Mustang. Ignoring his wild antics as he ran, scooted, and paced in the round pen, I remained outside the panels and huffed three soft breaths toward him as a general greeting. Timmy became irate, and pinned his ears, moving away from me.

Interesting.

So, I went to work, kicking the round pen panels, banging on the bark of a nearby tree, and tossing some rocks into the surrounding bushes. After about three minutes, Timmy stopped running and stood perfectly still, staring at me. I looked at him, and offered three huffing breaths again (soft, huffing breaths are an invitation to connect—see p. 40 to revisit Breath Messages).

Timmy flattened his ears again—but also looked away. In Horse Speak, looking away is considered very polite. Remember, horses use space like money; if they give a little space they are giving it *to you*. I acknowledged his gift of head space by taking one step back, and turning my own head away. This said, "Thank you for the room. Here is some for you."

Then I went back to tossing stones and ignoring him. In this way, I was not making the relationship with him primary. I was making the safeness of the environment primary and Timmy's presence in it secondary. I was "in charge" simply through my focus of attention on security.

It worked. Timmy dropped his head to the ground, sniffing the dirt in "Aw-Shucks." This meant "I want to take the pressure off," or it was a respectful request to get closer. Once again, I offered three huffing breaths and adopted an "O" posture with my arms in front of my body as I lightly bent forward. I was giving him the universal sign of welcome.

Timmy sauntered over to the edge of the round pen with soft eyes, but they were tented in worry. His chin was puckered with tension, but his nostrils were flaring, breathing me in. I held out my closed fist, knuckles up, toward his muzzle.

Horses greet each other in sets of three. The characteristics of the set of three can vary, depending on the horses involved. Timmy wanted to do fast, breathy touches on my knuckles, which I found to be typical for an uptight gelding. Males who have more of a "rough-housing" attitude will do three fast nostril flares upon reaching each other's muzzles. Horses who know each other well will do their greeting touches slowly, taking time between each one. Horses who are sorting out hierarchy may extend the process and perform three sets of three.

I wanted to act like a Mentor to Timmy, so I did one touch with my knuckles to his nose, but I requested we proceed from there more slowly than he wanted to. I didn't want to let him control the speed of our greeting, so I slowed it way down. Occasionally, when a horse is a bit uptight or anxious, I will allow a much faster greeting to happen at first, but I will return to it again later to have a nice, slow discussion.

Between each touch to Timmy's nose, I looked away as though some bogeyman had appeared on the horizon. I learned to do this by watching Sentry horses schooling younger or nervous herdmates: The Sentry would "scan the horizon" for danger to help calm them down. The methods the Mentor horse uses in this situation are pretty much the same, and that remains true whether the Mentor is a mare, gelding, or even a stallion.

Rule number one for Horse Speak: Go slowly; breathe a lot.

After I touched Timmy for the second muzzle greeting, he stepped away. In the three touches horses use to complete their conversation about hierarchy, leadership, safety, and connection, each stage is a chance to size the other horse up. The one who scans the horizon for bogeymen is the one who offers to lead. If a horse steps away on the second touch, he is not ready for a more intimate connection. Touch number three is a commitment, and Timmy was not ready for that.

I stepped back as well, and blew out a long sigh. I looked down at the ground, and Timmy lowered his head. I gazed at his tense eyes and blinked. Mentors use blinking to convince nervous horses there is nothing scary to stare at. Blinking can also indicate inner Zero, and horses use this to say they are so content and comfortable they wish to take a nap (a favorite discussion!).

After blinking back at me, Timmy blew out a long sigh and cleared his nose. This meant he was making a fresh start. He came right over to me and touched my hand for the third time, lingering and lipping my knuckles affectionately.

Lipping means the horse wants closeness. Given that Timmy was so volatile, I was not going to offer touch in return. As previously discussed, horses do not groom each other until all is safe, the relationship is on an even keel, their bellies are full, and nothing could be better than a little scratch. Touch is not high on *their* list of priorities—it is high on *our* list. Timmy knew this and was telling me I could go ahead and "invade" his space now. But I wanted to show him that I was not going to invade his space. By doing so I was able to tell him he couldn't invade mine, either. Establishing this mutual respect would go further than anything else I could do.

To emphasize our space negotiation, I aimed my pointer finger at his "Go Away Face" Button (under the eye on the round part of his cheek—see p. 42). I did not put my hand through the fence to touch this Button directly—I only needed to hold my pointer finger in position, aiming at the Button, for 30 seconds or so before he politely moved his face to the side.

Now I really had his attention.

Timmy came back and wanted what I call a "Check-In" knuckle touch right away. The Check-In is a soft, muzzle-to-knuckle touch that horses use on each other to simply connect. They can touch muzzle to muzzle or along any part of the body, or even just aim the muzzle from a distance. Between humans and horses, the muzzle-to-knuckle Check-In is reassuring and inspires bonding while still respecting personal space.

As soon as he did a Check-In, I asked Timmy for Go Away Face again. He gladly complied. We did this all over again, three more times. On the fourth time, he moved his whole head and neck away, and left it to the side while watching me out the corner of his eye. He was motionless. I complimented him out loud and softly stepped to the side as well, giving him the biggest "YES" I could: space and breath.

Timmy commenced then to yawn repeatedly. He released so much tension that his eyes rolled up in his head. I nodded my head at him to agree, and then lightly wiggled my lips while shaking my head side to side. He shook his head side to side, too, and wiggled his lips back. This meant he also felt like he was having a nice day. We no longer needed to be on edge with each other, and as his new leader, I requested we take a nap.

We stood still for about a full minute, and then I told Dave to walk away from the round pen with me as we allowed Timmy to soak up all that had taken place.

I had all the information I needed about what was troubling the Mustang.

It's All About Your Face

If you are not sure what your horse is saying through his facial expressions, copy his expression! Horses and humans have prehensile lips and many muscles in our faces. We, in fact, make similar expressions for similar reasons.

Humans often have tense faces around horses. When you concentrate, your mouth gets tight, your chin puckers, your eyes bulge, and you hold your breath. In Horse Speak, these same characteristics can be seen when one horse is displeased and is saying he might bite if the other horse doesn't get a move on.

Humans look like "biters" most of the time, so horses must look for other clues as to what we want. As soon as humans start softening up their lips, eyes, and expressions, horses become interested, and feel much more comfortable.

"X," "O," and Thought Control

Since it is not always possible to monitor all our thoughts, developing the habit of softening our eyes, lips, and posture (creating the physical "O" that helps create the internal Zero) is a shortcut to making certain we are able to express and maintain a peaceful demeanor.

Horses do, at times, require an "X" posture. In an "X," our arms and legs move out firmly and our intensity becomes higher. We make an "X" to create motivation to move, to block against movement, or to simply signal intention. Horses are not intrinsically afraid of an "X" posture, but they do fear a person who is stuck in "X." Many people find it difficult to modulate their own intensity, and what should simply be assertive often becomes aggressive. In an effort to help make this clear, I usually teach people to think of levels of intensity in five layers: *Zero, intention, asking, telling*, and finally *insisting*.

- Level One intensity occurs simply by looking with purpose at a Button, as opposed to casually blinking your eyes while at Zero.

- Level Two is the first request for a Button to do something (this could be a request to hold still, come to you, or move away from you). This level of intensity is about as much pressure as you would use while holding the hand of a toddler: not much and very gentle.

- Level Three happens when you really need a horse to "do the thing," and he doesn't seem to desire to. This can include sliding your hand down a lead rope and giving it a "scoop," or using a bit more pressure in your touch, or adding a little noise like snapping fingers or clucking. (I find people cluck way too often and too much, so I like to use finger snapping, because you have to be deliberate to do it.)

- Level Four intensity happens when you really, really need a horse to "do the thing," and he really, really doesn't want to. However, this level of intensity also occurs when horses show off for each other, like during a big play session. To avoid going overboard, I have come up with strategies to help people develop a safe and sane Level Four that horses believe, and better still, that will not offend them. In fact, at the very beginning of working with a new horse when I "scan the horizon" or "secure the environment," I am at a Level Four *for the horse's sake*. I am showing him that I can mean business about the big, scary world. I do not want to get confrontational with a horse, so by acting like a strong Leader (based on the model of the Mother), and checking out all the bogeymen, I am less likely to need to go beyond a Level Three when we start working more closely with each other. I have already psychologically established myself as capable of a Level Four. Horses sometimes *want* to see our Level Four because it makes them feel secure; ironically, this is especially true for horses that have had poor handling. The mistake people most often make is that we can perpetuate their fear by reacting with aggression rather than assertiveness. I have specific exercises to help students learn the difference, because in our culture, the two are often confused. (In the horse world, assertive can be at a high intensity, but as soon as it's over, it's over…and everyone takes a nap!)

Most people do not want to live aggressively with their horses, and so in the effort to avoid this complication, they undercut their "X" energy. In other words, a person may be saying, "Go," or "Stop," and making the right noises or motions, yet underneath it all she doesn't really want the horse to feel offended, or she is afraid to accidentally ruin the connection she feels she has with her horse.

"Boundary" is not a four-letter word. It does not imply punishment, restriction of authenticity, or rigidity.

Horses need sane, healthy boundaries much like the two sides of a river. If the shores of a river are too muddy, the river merges with the land and it all becomes swamp. Horses thrive on clear boundaries amongst themselves. The cohesiveness of their life together depends upon their ability to move their large bodies deftly around each other. In the case of a crisis, this ability means all the horses can run at top speed and not trip each other up. Roads have lines so we do not drive across them and into each other. For a prey animal, boundaries are the edges of their private and personal space—the line in the road to be crossed with care.

To maintain healthy assertiveness, we need to think of the edges of our boundaries like the bowl we would pour soup into. If the bowl has cracks in it, the soup will run out. If the soup represents the nourishing parts of your relationship with your horse, then you can see it is imperative to have clean, healthy boundaries so that both horse and human have the nourishment they need.

Healthy horses thrive on tidy assertiveness that does not take much time or energy. I call this "low calorie conversation." If a horse raises his head, puts his ears back, and tightens his lips while aiming his eyes at the "Go Away Face" button on another horse's cheek, he only needs the other horse to move his face away a bit. Horses have long necks and heads, and it is considered polite to simply move a head away from the space of a higher herd member. Moving the feet may not be required, unless the higher-ranked member wants to take over the space the lower member is currently in.

Keeping this in mind, you can begin to see that maintaining an "O" posture and a level Zero internally is the basis for maintaining the peace between requests. Horses make requests of each other all the time, and by keeping their head lowered, ears sideways, eyes soft, lips and chin relaxed, they are using the horse version of "O" posture and maintaining a Zero inner energy. Starting at Zero, you might ask for Go Away Face, then return to Zero when it is complied with. If the horse is confused by this, thinking that your Zero is also an "O" that is welcoming him to return, he may quickly come back into your space. In this case, you may need to establish that boundary: hold a constant "X" posture, but the secret is to never leave Zero internally. Your goal is to clear up confusion, not adopt a negative attitude.

By having the foundation be Zero, it is easier and easier for smaller and smaller versions of "X" to serve as boundaries. Horses are actually masters at the lowest level "X" messages. Most of us have seen a lead horse that rarely even lifts his head—his eyes alone are his "X."

Because humans tend to merge their "Xs" and "Os" unconsciously, horses learn to tune us out. Then, we find ourselves having to amplify our "X" energy to a ridiculous level to be heard.

This was, unfortunately, Timmy's problem.

Timmy Finds His Zero

I asked Dave to halter Timmy and show me some of the groundwork he was doing with his horse. Although on the surface Dave and Timmy certainly knew the exercises they were doing together, a few things became clear to me.

After watching Dave catch, halter, and lead Timmy, I could see that he was a cheery, light-hearted guy who loved his horse…but became stiff and defensive around him. This was understandable, because the moment Dave began leading the Mustang, Timmy began to attempt to chew on Dave. The horse wasn't being completely offensive or dangerous in his behavior—instead it came across like a game that went kind of like this:

Timmy: "I want to chew on your arm."

Dave: "No, Timmy…. No, Timmy…. C'mon, Timmy. Cut it out, Timmy…. NO, TIMMY!"

Timmy: "Hmmpf! FINE!!!"

Timmy then pouted with wrinkled eyes and a tense mouth for about a minute, before sneaking in another attempt to chew on Dave.

What I could see was that while Dave certainly didn't want his horse nibbling on him, he didn't *entirely* mind that his horse wanted to play. His "X" and "O" were blurred, and the soup was leaking from the bowl.

What I had gathered in my earlier conversation with Dave was that at some point in their round pen sessions, Timmy tended to settle down. This told me Dave eventually became enough of a believable "X" that Timmy felt reassured about where his place was. When Dave's "X" was strong enough, Timmy's behavior improved. I now needed to ask Dave a question.

"Dave, you don't really like having to constantly tell him to cut it out, do you?" I asked bluntly.

"No," he admitted. And then, "But I don't want to hurt his feelings. I have had this guy since he was a few months old, and sometimes when I put him in his place, it seems like then he won't even come to me after. I want him to trust me. I need him to know that I would never hurt him. My trainer tells me I must get tougher with him—but not angry. Honestly, I don't see the difference between 'tough' and 'angry.' And sometimes Timmy is so much to handle that I *do* get angry; then I really feel bad."

AHA MOMENT

It was a swamp, all right. Timmy was acting out the same way a human toddler does who needs both boundaries and enough room to say, "I can do it *myself.*"

One side of Timmy's river was allowing him to be responsible for holding down his own set of healthy boundaries. The other side of the river was Dave's ability to find the delicate balance between friendship with his buddy and mentorship with his student.

I said to Dave, "Do you think Timmy's mother would have allowed him to chew on her whenever he wanted?"

Dave's eyes brightened as he replied, "I got to see him with his mom for a few days at the auction. She was cool as a cucumber with him, and he did *not* chew on her. I did see her licking his head, though. Come to think of it, it always made me feel sad that he was taken away from her, and I think I felt like I had to make up for that loss. But…that's just how things were done at the Mustang auction."

It was now pretty darn clear to me as to how and why this relationship got so muddy.

I told Dave that I was going to work with him to learn to feel the difference in his body between "aggressive" or "angry energy" and simple, assertive, clear, "'X' energy." I explained that Timmy's mom had been clear and simple with him, and that is why she was able to give her baby affection and not have him get out of control. I also told Dave that it was time to give Timmy the right to grow up instead of remaining the baby in Dave's sad memory.

Dave wanted Timmy to behave himself, but his baggage had weighed down the relationship. Dave and I worked on some exercises to help him find the power of assertiveness without any baggage. I made different levels of "X" postures and gestures toward Dave, and he told me which ones were aggressive and which ones were polite but assertive. I explained that since he was offering to be his horse's leader, he needed to be the model of behavior he would like the horse to copy. If we are flailing and inconsistent, then that is what we tell the horse to be, too. If we are rigid and inflexible, then that is the message.

I helped Dave find and maintain his Zero and "O" posture, then do something engaging like throw a stone, but coming right back to Zero. Dave was surprised at how hard it was to return to Zero after raising up his adrenaline when he aimed and threw a rock toward a nearby tree. I explained that this was how he found himself in the "never-ending 'X'" that horses find difficult—there wasn't a "real" Zero for Dave to rely on. I believed that since Dave didn't want to come across like a bully and was afraid of hurting his horse's feelings, he was too passive, *but* his passive energy was not Zero, either! He needed to solve the riddle of how to stay firm on one hand, but loving and open on the other.

Suddenly, it dawned on Dave that he might have his own solution. He had studied martial arts for many years, and he told me about how he'd learned to make a "Ki-aye!" sound when hitting a board, for instance. His teacher had said this released all the stored power into the punch and freed the person from residual tension so that he returned to a state of calm.

Ki-Aye

A big smile widened across my face.

"Dave, you are going to 'Ki-aye' near Timmy so that he can hear and see you."

At first, Dave was concerned that this would upset Timmy. I assured him that this demonstration of power *with immediate return to Zero* was exactly what his horse was looking for.

We went inside Timmy's paddock, and the horse looked up from his hay but did not come over. I had Dave aim at the side of the round pen and pretend to hit one of the panels (we didn't want to *actually* break anything). Timmy became very, very still, staring at Dave, who stood where he was, practicing his martial arts breathing with palms down toward the earth to ground himself.

Timmy then offered a very clear Go Away Face and moved his neck to the side, too, holding this posture for a good minute. Dave was blown away—was Timmy deferring space to him? Then he remembered that he had actually seen Timmy do this on several occasions, only he had always thought it meant the horse was tuning him out.

When Timmy brought his face back around to look at Dave, it was no longer wrinkled around his eyes and his ears had flopped to the sides. He bobbed his head and then did an "Aw-Shucks" to show he wanted to keep the energy calm and respectful. I told Dave to do the same thing, nodding his head, and scuffing the ground lightly with the toe of his boot. Then I had Dave turn slightly to the side to invite Timmy to his shoulder—where horses line up for bonding.

Timmy made a beeline for Dave's shoulder, stopping just outside his bubble of personal space for one more head turn and Aw-Shucks to make sure he was welcome, and that the energy was just right for them both. The Mustang then reached over while elongating his neck in a proper, polite, horse greeting and touched Dave's knuckles lightly with his lips.

Dave smiled ear to ear.

But then his eagerness overcame him, and he reached through both of their "bubbles of personal space" to rub Timmy on the head.

Timmy immediately pulled back, pinned his ears, and puckered up his whole face in what could be described as disgust. Then he reached over and nipped Dave's arm before marching away.

I didn't need to say a thing. Dave's eyes had grown wide and he pronounced loudly, "I totally blew it, didn't I?"

Dave had gotten the first glimpse of what Timmy's problem really was: He was extremely protective of his personal space, and in Dave's attempt to be extra friendly with him, Dave unintentionally caused his horse to feel invaded. Another horse that was more stoic would have probably just come to ignore Dave's loving and learned to take it in stride, but Timmy was wild-born. Personal space was always going to be important to him.

I went back to the drawing board with Dave. We practiced his "Ki-aye" intensity, with the ability to stay at or return to Zero becoming more and more attainable. I also taught Dave to imagine a glass wall between us that we would literally bump into when moving through the exercises. I had Dave hold his hand out at arm's length like a cop stopping traffic whenever I tried to get too close to him. He did not need to stop me physically or yell at me—he simply had to let me know where his glass wall was, always.

Next I helped him become aware of his bellybutton. Why? Because where we aim our bellybutton is where we aim to go. We can be looking left, but if our bellybutton is aiming right, that is where we are going to end up. Horses know this. For them this directive center is their chest. Wherever their chest is aiming tells you where they truly intend to move. I had Dave keep his "cop-stop" hand at his bellybutton to help illustrate how he could maintain his "bubble of space." By learning to keep his own "bubble" defined, he would make Timmy's more defined. The security Timmy would feel from this would be the soothing balm that would lead to a truly authentic connection between Timmy and Dave. When this happened, natural affection such as what the Mustang's mother had given him would be allowed to emerge.

Round Three

With a big breath, Dave entered Timmy's pen again. He nodded his head, turned a little to the side, aiming his shoulder at his horse, and held out his knuckles. Then Dave bent over just a little to make more of an "O" and welcome Timmy to his side. Timmy wasted no time, walking over with a lowered head, sideways ears, and a lot of huffing breaths coming out of his nostrils. Timmy was using a beckoning expression to tell Dave that he wanted to try again, too.

They had one, two, three touches softly and quickly but not the speed-racer version Timmy had offered me at the beginning of the day. The Mustang wanted all three touches from Dave to symbolize an official greeting in which all the rules were followed. This was very, very good. If Timmy followed the horse rules of conduct, and Dave followed the rules, too, the outcome for them together would be much better.

Timmy then offered Go Away Face, which he dramatically performed and held for about 30 seconds. I told Dave to mimic this, moving his head away a bit, to say, "Thank you. Very good." The Mustang politely reached for Dave's knuckles to perform a Check-In. He was seeking connection and security, as he would with another horse with whom he'd bonded. Dave lingered while breathing deeply, then moved his hand away. This was done perfectly, and Timmy, again, offered Go Away Face to show his respect for Dave's personal space. I instructed Dave to take one defined, clear step away from his horse to indicate he was more concerned about personal space than contact right now. Timmy took one, dramatic step away from Dave, too. I call this "Copycat."

Now I had Dave initiate a Check-In, immediately followed by pointing toward the Go Away Face Button so that he could begin to demonstrate his role as leader. Dave did this very clearly and cleanly, and Timmy not only did Go Away Face but took his whole body in a circle and then came back to greet Dave one more time. I told Dave that this was Timmy's way of saying he trusted him with all his body parts, all his Buttons, and in fact his whole self. When a horse offers this polite "Sail-By" movement that is performed slowly and deliberately, he is saying he trusts you to not be a Bully, and that you are welcome to move any part of him. Timmy not only did a Sail-By, he also circled and came back. This meant he understood that he and Dave were bonded, and he should return to him.

Dave admitted that during this sequence his mind had been doubtful, and the voice in his head had been saying things like, "See, he's leaving you…. This isn't working…. He's ignoring you…" Yet the feeling he had when Timmy turned and came back was one of such warmth and happiness.

Dave's worst fear was that by setting limits, he would lose Timmy's affection, and possibly be betraying his trust. However, the consequences of not setting clean, low-intensity boundaries had been to make Timmy feel frantic, overwhelmed, and nippy. Helping Dave find ways to set boundaries using Horse Speak gave him tools to try that were within reason, and safe, for both of them.

Cooking Class

The difference between training and communicating can be best illustrated with a cooking class metaphor. Let's say you want to learn to make a real Italian lasagna, and you sign up for a cooking class with that goal in mind. You have a huge smile on your face as you enter the classroom full of delicious smells. You've never been so excited to learn something new! As you find a seat next to another student, your instructor turns to the class and says, "Ciao!" and proceeds to speak in Italian.

Let's suppose you do not know Italian, but many of the students do, and so a lovely conversation in another language is flying around the room as the instruments are pulled out and the various foods are diced, boiled, chopped, and sautéed.

At the end of class, you have followed along enough to be able to pull something out of the oven. Yours does not look like the others, but it smells okay and you think you more or less got the gist of it. Yet the class was confusing, and you felt left out of all the jokes, and frustrated that you couldn't even ask a simple question.

Welcome to a horse's life.

Horses do not speak human, although many learn enough to get by. Whatever the horse *has* come to learn about what we expect from him, the desired outcome, the "why," and the reasons behind the "why," are a mystery to him. If, by chance, he discovers a method to our madness, and starts to predict what we want, he may be chastised for "anticipating." He is often confused, rarely gets the jokes, and usually can't communicate his questions.

All the while, maybe the horse doesn't even like lasagna!

The main objective of the cooking class was to learn to make food, but the class itself was about socializing, communicating, bonding, and togetherness… all of which were only possible if you could speak the language. And what if someone in the class borrowed all your implements, slopped their chopped garlic all over your part of the counter, and spilled wine on your apron? Not only would you be frustrated by your inability to point out how rude he was being, you might even want to hit (or bite!) him.

Horse Speak is about learning the language so that the bridge of understanding can be crossed. Once horses know you are trying to talk to them—even if your accent is thick—they immediately try to reach back across that bridge to talk to you, too.

Timmy and Dave Bake Lasagna

Timmy and Dave were off to a new beginning, but there were a few more aspects of communication we needed to introduce to help their relationship progress.

In all their years together, haltering had been a huge drag, according to Dave, with Timmy pinning his ears and evading. There is often confusion related to haltering, so I had Dave and Timmy try an exercise called "Say Hello to Your Halter": three touches to the halter and Go Away Face (in which both Timmy and the halter moved away to show respect from both sides). Then I had Dave walk a small circle and return with the halter to show Timmy that he could trust him. Timmy bowed his head low, blew through his nose profusely, licked his lips, and blinked his eyes to loudly demonstrate agreement—and a bit of a "Whew! Glad that's cleared up!"

Then Timmy stood stock still as Dave put on the halter *while keeping his bellybutton facing forward*, and aiming his shoulder at the Mustang's shoulder. Basically, they were both facing the same direction, with Dave a little further back than he would be usually. The big difference, however, was that normally, Dave *faced* his horse, and his bellybutton (and probably some "X") was a driving pressure that Timmy wanted to scoot away from.

I had them repeat the exercise several times. By the end, Dave walked slowly around the pen holding the halter, with Timmy following the halter as though he was enamored of it! The last time Dave stepped up with the halter raised, the horse practically stuck it on his own face. Dave was smiling ear to ear and shaking his head.

Now it was time to practice leading Timmy from the perspective of body language.

When we are babies, and we first learn to crawl, we place our palms down to do so. Our brains are hard-wired to feel grounded when we hold our palms downward. This message can be directly sent through the lead rope to a horse, if you are willing give up holding the lead rope in the usual fashion with your hand closest to the horse's head "thumb-up." Most people don't actually give this much thought—they simply grab the rope as it hangs from the halter and walk forward. This seems logical enough, however, when we grab onto something with our thumb up, we are using muscle (mostly bicep) to move whatever it is. This works well for paddling a canoe or digging a ditch, but not so much for encouraging a horse to follow us softly.

I demonstrated: I had Dave hold the clasp of the lead rope in two hands out in front of him at arm's length. The rope fell naturally downward, as it would if the clasp was attached to the bottom ring of a halter. I took the rope in my hand with my thumb *up* as most of us would normally do, and motioned for him to follow. Placing a tiny amount of pressure on the rope to let the horse (in this case, Dave) know he should come forward (again as most of us would do), I watched as Dave's upper body reacted to the sudden perceived tug. He lurched forward a step, with his eyes wide in surprise, then his face hardened, as he took stubborn, rigid steps.

I then proceeded to try to make a sharp turn like anyone might do to close a gate or a stall door. Dave slammed into me, and I used my elbow defensively (as we often do with our horses) to keep him from toppling over onto me. Dave acknowledged the "elbow thing" was far too familiar to him.

After shaking that off for a minute, we started again. I had him resume holding the clasp of the lead rope out in front, and this time I exaggerated rounding my arm over and downward to demonstrate the way to place your palm downward onto the lead rope with your pinky finger facing upward, and your thumb pointed downward. As you move to lead forward and your hand rises, your knuckles are in the same position that they are for saying "Hello" or doing a Check-In… and so you may find your horse wants to—a huge benefit because it encourages bonding and responsiveness to you as a kind leader that your horse *wants* to follow. In addition, when a horse has a habit of being defensive and nippy when led, you can simply raise your lead rope knuckles up toward the Go Away Face Button and even point your finger at it as you walk along. If necessary, you can lead the horse the whole way in this position, which simply says to him, "Let's have space the *whole time* we are going somewhere together." Generally, horses that are nippy while being lead simply feel too close to their handlers or like their space has been invaded—or they are confused about what is too close or not close enough. Your palm down on the lead rope offers a stabilizing sensation to the horse.

Dave was amazed as now we waltzed along in perfect harmony; he found himself happy to walk in step and even halt in time with me. But, he wondered, what should he do about when Timmy "got stubborn"?

With a smile, I asked him to resist me. He was a big man, and as he leaned back against the lead rope, I performed the "scooping-up" motion I'd discovered with Rocky (see p. 80). With my hand in the same palm-down position, I rotated my whole arm as though scooping a huge round of ice cream out of one of those big bins at the ice cream parlor—then I just stood there. After about 30 seconds, the weight and tension he was applying to the lead rope eased, and I immediately released the "scoop" like it was a hot potato. Then I "scooped" one more time, and Dave found himself willingly following the motion before he could even think about it. I returned my hand to a palm-down position and let out some slack in the rope so he could have more room. He found himself drifting comfortably to the side of me, and I elevated my arm and hand out to my side an extra 4 inches. Like the "cop-stop" hand from before, only with a palm-down invitation to keep moving, I was defining my "bubble" but welcoming him to follow.

Eager to try the leading technique with Timmy, Dave re-entered the round pen, and Timmy immediately sauntered over. Dave said hello and blew a long, slow breath at Timmy to show connection. Timmy blew back, and lowered his head. Dave slipped the halter on without a problem and clipped on the lead rope. Timmy's head shot up, and a worried look came over him. I told Dave that "the only way through was through," and he should start leading his horse. After he took a few nervous steps, I told Dave to aim his palm-down hand toward Timmy's Go Away Face Button and give the Mustang some slack in the rope. In about two strides, Timmy blew out a huge breath of relief and shook his head like a dog shaking the water of his coat after a bath. His head dropped lower, and his ears flopped sideways. I encouraged the pair to walk around obstacles in the pen and change directions a few times. I reminded Dave to make one clear stomp when he wanted to stop because horses lead through their feet and stop each other that way, too. Timmy halted on a dime, lining up his front feet with Dave's.

Going Back to Go Forward

Dave led Timmy out of the pen and around the surrounding area. A few times, Timmy became nervous and attempted to herd Dave back toward the pen, but Dave now raised his "X" an appropriate amount (managing his power like his "Ki-aye") and easily redirected Timmy using the Mid-Neck and Shoulder Buttons (p. 42). He also practiced something I call the "Therapy Back-Up" whenever Timmy became pushy. This specific movement releases tension in the lower back and pelvis of the horse, which is why I call it "therapeutic." Horses tuck their tails when nervous, like dogs, and their pelvis can store quite a lot of habitual tension. By releasing this tension, we also encourage the horse to release stored anxiety or fear.

The first time I helped Dave into position to work the Therapy Back-Up, Timmy resisted, swishing his tail and lifting his chest up in complaint. I told Dave to keep his eyes on Timmy's rump, while tickling the Back-Up Button (located at the apex of the triangle shape exactly where the front leg meets the bulk of the shoulder—see p. 42). As soon as Dave touched the Button, Timmy's whole front leg shook in a spasm. This spot is full of nerves, which is why you only need to point at it to have an effect. Dave practiced a "reverse scoop" under Timmy's chin, drawing toward his chest. The whole effect was to encourage the horse's skeleton to round and release. Dave was amazed as we literally saw Timmy's hind end buckle and soften downward. He asked for a single step back (this should feel good to the horse, not like you are being pushy). They did one step at a time, with pauses in between, for a few minutes until Timmy suddenly began to yawn profusely. I told Dave to step to the Mustang's shoulder, keeping his bellybutton angled away from his horse, to take any pressure off him and encourage even more relaxation.

When they stepped forward again to resume their walk, Timmy had dropped his head, neck, and shoulders, as well as any tension in his belly. Essentially, he looked shorter and fatter. He was blinking his eyes and taking huge breaths.

Finally, it was time to show real affection. We brought Timmy back into the round pen, and turned him loose. I explained that horses only enjoy affection with each other when all the other aspects of their relationship are settled and the world is safe.

Dave nodded his head slightly to let Timmy know he wanted to get closer. Timmy moved his head and neck to the side and "popped" his shoulder toward Dave, telling him to "buddy up." Dave went to the horse's shoulder and began to stroke his withers in a soothing, downward motion. (Scratching with an up-and-down motion might feel good to the horse, but it goes against the growth of the hair and can be overstimulating.) Gently rocking his own body while he did this, Dave soon found that Timmy had lowered his head and was yawning so wide that his eyes were rolling back in his head. I had Dave move toward Timmy's head—about two small steps forward—while trailing his hand forward through his horse's mane. When Dave's hand reached the back of Timmy's poll, the Mustang dropped his head even lower and flopped his ears sideways. I told Dave he could run his hand firmly but gently between the horse's ears and onto his forehead. Timmy pressed his head close to Dave's body while Dave stroked him. I encouraged Dave to lightly roll his hands over Timmy's eyes while thinking how he wanted his horse to close his eyes and trust him. Timmy loved this so much that he gently moved his head into Dave's hands even more.

It is important not to be greedy in these moments. I let Dave know it was time to quietly step away. Timmy just gazed at the big man as though he had been drugged. Then, he pawed the ground and laid down!

So we just hung out, quietly talking about Dave's experience while standing guard over the deeply peaceful Timmy.

Dave felt guilty for not understanding his horse's true needs before. He knew his regular trainer meant well…but fundamentally Dave had not understood the intentions and meanings behind his horse's reactions and messages, and how the work he did with him influenced this behavior.

Horses forgive much more quickly than we do. All Timmy cared about was that Dave would be consistent now that they had found a better platform for their relationship.

As he stood in quiet reflection, Dave admitted that the encounter he had just experienced reminded him of the deep love he witnessed Timmy sharing with his mom. He was supremely happy to have finally reached that level of connection with his horse—this had been his goal all along, and the force behind whatever other training technique Dave tried to use.

Transitions

After this pivotal experience, Dave felt much more confident about the other aspects of the "work" he liked to do with his horse. They enjoyed trail riding together, and Dave aspired to do Western Dressage. Under saddle, Timmy was pretty good, but they did have "arguments" from time to time. With his new-found understanding, those arguments were replaying in Dave's mind in a whole new light—he now felt he had some idea of what may have been bothering his horse at those times.

I told Dave that the next time he and Timmy entered the round pen to practice transitions before he got on, he needed to have *exactly* what he wanted to do in mind. I even had him write it down: "Timmy, we are going into the round pen to practice transitions and get ready for riding. This is supposed to be fun, and I am here for you. Don't worry about a thing."

The problem was not necessarily the transition work in the round pen, but the lack of connection to each other while doing it. Trotting and cantering around was not going to magically make a relationship happen nor would it suddenly make Timmy feel or act safe. Dave had been so stuck in his own feelings—sadness and guilt for the way his horse lost his life in the wild and then his mother—that putting Timmy through his paces was not actually fun for him. He had only done it because otherwise he did not feel he could trust his horse under saddle.

Giving Dave a new way of thinking about staying connected even while working in the round pen was the missing link.

I felt confident that they would be able to work through any future confusion now that Dave was aware and open to his horse's means of communicating. The fact that we had arrived at such an affectionate and lovely moment between the two of them ensured that he too saw the value of understanding how his horse saw him, as well as how his horse related to the world.

Lick and Chew

On the list of top 10 things that are misunderstood between horses and people, I would say that *healthy boundaries* are near the top. Perhaps it is because of our tendency to look at horses and wish for puppy piles, or it is due to our habit of relating to an idea inside our own heads instead of seeing what is right in front of us.

For far too many people, healthy boundaries are a challenge in life for any number of reasons. Horses offer us the chance to work out this confusion in a spirit of connection. They need and want us to be simple, quiet, and clear about our "bubbles" of personal space *before* we start merging them. The Go Away Face Button is the cleanest, calmest, and most direct Button horses possess for this very reason. Although this can seem too easy, sometimes Horse Speak really is that simple.

Once we understand that a horse turning his head calmly away from us (or even stepping gently away) is a compliment, and that horses use space like a commodity, so much clarity can come to light. Even if a horse has turned away and doesn't seem to want to engage, the very act of turning away means that he has yielded the space to you. He may not want to hang out with you right now, but he didn't drive you off, he gave you room. We ruin the possibility for peaceful connection when we take this personally and go after him.

Everyone needs clear "Xs" and "Os"— not merging, confusing signals. The bonding is always better as soon as boundaries are cleared up.

And remember, to truly communicate clearly with a horse, we must understand what dark thoughts may be lurking in the back of our own minds. Like a horse gives us space, we must be able to give those dark thoughts some space. Only then can we truly reach out for connection.

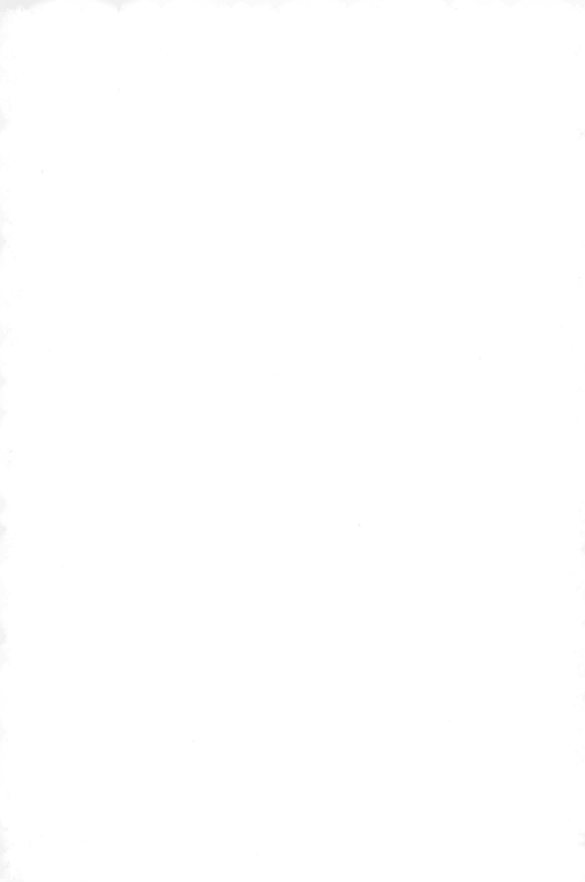

Chapter 8

The Horse on the Hill

Mist in the Trees

A rescue contacted me about a horse that wouldn't be caught.

When I arrived at the farm, I was greeted by a cheery, middle-aged woman I'll call "Rosa." She had started the rescue several years before when she discovered that a horse she had once sold had died of starvation when the police were given a tip and the barn where the horse had been living was raided. There were many sad cases that day, but for Rosa the horror of the death of a horse that had once been her own was close, cutting, and personal.

Rosa had managed to help over a hundred "rescue" horses find loving new homes since then. Some came from auctions, some from families who fell on hard times and couldn't afford the costs of care anymore, and some came from terrible, unhappy places.

The horse I was being asked to help was one from a more unfortunate situation. The history Rosa knew of was bad: The last person to have owned him had been running a questionable trail riding outfit where the horses were kept locked up in filthy stalls all day and night between rides, and this horse apparently hadn't left his stall at all for several weeks due to an infection in his leg. He had not had his feet trimmed in many months, the leg infection was oozing, and he was extremely underweight.

Rosa called him Marty, and he was a big gray that looked like some sort of Percheron cross. Marty was quiet and kind-hearted, but everyone who worked with him during his first few months as he was nursed back to health came away with an overwhelming sense of sadness.

Finally, when Marty had healed enough, he was let out on pasture with other geldings at the rescue. That, however, was the last time *anyone* had been able to touch him. Reveling in his newfound freedom, Marty had no intention of ever coming down off the side of the mountain he now called home. Rosa left food and water for him near the gate, and every morning and evening the food would be gone…but Marty would not even come in close if she or another human was anywhere near during these "feeding times."

The last thing Rosa wanted to do was chase him around or force him to be caught—for obvious reasons—yet he needed to have his hooves trimmed and his still healing leg wound was due to be checked by a vet. One volunteer had spent a whole day patiently trying to get close to him, with no luck. Another had offered to ride a horse out in the field and try to rope him. Rosa could not imagine the big horse being roped without it being traumatic, but she did feel her options were few.

Marty was in a large pasture that included a steep incline up the side of a mountain. All the other geldings were at the bottom of the hill. Up in the tree line, I caught a glimpse of the big gray, moving like mist in the forest.

I surveyed the motions of the herd. There was one horse, a big chestnut, that stood with his face aimed in my direction, and although he was eating grass he was staring right at me. He was positioned at the head of the herd, with the others fanned out like a flock of geese behind him. Rosa said his name was "Red."

This was the horse I needed to talk to.

Big Red

Rosa and I, along with two volunteers who wanted to observe, went inside the pasture. As a precaution, I had a cotton lead rope coiled and tucked into my back pocket. I had never met this group of horses, and while Rosa said they were all nice, you never know what can happen. The rope was my emergency "send away" tool that could act as an extension of my arm, should I need it. I never walk into a pen or pasture with horses I don't know with a flag, crop, whip, or other training stick because you never know how a horse will react to a person with one of these tools. A length of rope is, however, a reasonable safety item.

I inspected the ground, the gate, and the water trough as though the herd of geldings didn't even exist. This got the chestnut's attention.

I then sauntered off to the left a few feet, inspecting the trees in that direction. Licking my lips, I turned around, sauntered off to the right, and inspected those trees. Last, I walked three steps toward Red, cocked my hip, and dug my toe into the ground while sighing loudly.

I had said, "Hmmmm…nothing bad to the left. Nothing bad to the right. Nothing seems bad about you. I think I will stay right here and relax."

Red lifted his head and nodded a tiny bit. I nodded back at him and sighed again, scuffing my toe to tell him I had no agenda. Red looked left, then right, then down, then sauntered all the way over to me with a nice swinging step. When horses move with a good swing in their backs, they are saying, "There is no rush and nothing to worry about." If he had come toward me peg-legged and stiff with a high head, I would have made an "X" with my body to tell him to stop and gone back outside the gate for a moment before returning to try again after a pause. Usually, this is enough to tell a horse not to rush or approach me in an aggressive manner, and the second encounter is much calmer.

Red was already calm, so luckily, I didn't need to do anything but stay at Zero and sigh out a lot. I smiled and blinked as he approached, and he drooped his lower lip and blinked as well. The chestnut paused just outside my "bubble of personal space" to look left and right and down again. He was already telling me he agreed that there wasn't any reason for concern and we might have a nice day together.

I reached long and low, stretching my torso and arm outward toward his muzzle with my knuckles up. His first inclination was to lip my hand as though I might be holding a treat or cookie. Rosa said that she often gave cookies when catching the geldings to keep them happy and interested. They all had such checkered pasts, she just wanted to let them know they were treasured now.

I moved my knuckles away, and turned my head aside to the left to tell Red I was doing a real greeting, not giving cookies. He turned his head that way, too, to signal he would follow my lead.

Reaching in for the second touch, Red now politely touched the back of my hand ever so lightly. I straightened up, smiled, and nodded at him, and he turned in a lovely Go Away Face gesture to show respect.

I didn't need to wait at all for the third Greeting touch, as Red was already initiating it. On this one, we lingered, and I breathed long and softly toward his muzzle. He responded by widening his nostrils and inhaling my scent deeply.

This huffing breathing is how horses say, "I know you." A horse's unique scent is his or her name. I told him I "knew" him, too. The three touches had established that I could "speak horse," and that I was confident. He was confident, as well, which was why he was the leader of the gelding herd.

Rosa explained that Red had been a feral stallion once, and his whole band was rounded up and shot, while he had been kept due to his size and strength. He worked as a ranch horse for some time, but then was injured and eventually shipped to auction. He could do light riding now, and Rosa loved to go out on trails with him because he was so surefooted and smart.

Now that our greeting was complete, I asked Red to move his face away, which he did, then slowly moved his feet and turned his whole body in a smooth arc to saunter back to what he had been doing before I showed up. I waved my hand by my thigh to symbolize the tail swish that says, "I'm done," and he replied with a tail swish of his own.

The other horses had been watching, and now one by one, they moved a few steps toward me. I suggested to Rosa and the volunteers that we all go up to each gelding and touch knuckles to muzzles to say a formal hello to all of them. As we went through the herd, touching the muzzles of the eight horses, it was interesting to see that some wanted all three touches in a row, and some would do two, then turn away and not do a third...yet. I explained to my own little herd of humans that this was good information—each horse had a different comfort level; we shouldn't take anything personally.

Very quickly, the geldings perked up: Many blew out their noses, shook their heads, and had sideways ears. Some were blinking. All of them lowered their necks and shoulders, and relaxed their belly muscles. More than a few wiggled their lips. These were all messages about comfort, safety, and pleasure.

I explained how to use the Go Away Face Button when Rosa or the volunteers needed more space or were ready to move on. I told them to use their pointer finger to ask a horse to step aside and give space, as opposed to pressing a palm against the horse. To the horse, a pressed palm feels like an invitation to come closer. To demonstrate, I told Rosa to press her palm into Red's Go Away Face Button, and then retract her hand and take a step backward. As though he was on an invisible string, Red swung his noble head around toward her with an enamored look on his face. He moved right into her hands and she lovingly stroked his forehead.

AHA MOMENT

A light bulb had gone off inside everyone's head. They all wanted to try both the pointer finger and the palm on the Button. I explained that while this was a good idea, they had to be sure to pause between asking for two different things and return to Zero. Otherwise it would become blurred body language and the horses would get confused.

Rosa and each volunteer used the pointer finger first to signal the horse should give space, then stepped back and took a breath before stepping in again and using a palm press on the same Button. After the palm press, I told each person in the group to "scoop" her hand back toward her body, as though tugging on an invisible string.

Laughs of surprise and delight, as well as loud snorts and shakes of the head, were everywhere. Horse and human alike enjoyed this lovely encounter.

The two horses that had formerly held out for their third Greeting touch now came toward us and asked to complete the greeting. Everyone could feel a release of tension. It was like a wave of warmth sifted through all our bodies, leaving everyone in a state of grace.

As a group, we practiced moving in and out of each horse's "bubble of personal space." It can sometimes be hard to see where the imaginary "glass wall" is, and that can lead to us standing too close to a horse. You want to orient yourself toward the horse's shoulder—not his face. As I've mentioned, horses use their shoulders to buddy up and their faces to greet another or negotiate things. Once a greeting is over, remaining too close results in the same sort of uncomfortable feeling that you would get if a person stood much too close after shaking your hand.

I encouraged Rosa and the volunteers to aim their bodies in the same direction the horses were...so their bellybuttons were off the Buttons of the horse. Once in this more comfortable space, I encouraged them all to scratch each horse's itchy spots. One by one, the geldings carefully told us when they wanted to change position by first sniffing our feet or by moving their own foot clearly and loudly and slowly off to the side. In either case, the horse was broadcasting his intentions a full 30 seconds before he moved out of care for his companion's wellbeing. The more we as people try to move around horses with self-awareness and respect for "bubbles of personal space," the more the horses will, too.

Suddenly, as we were scratching and grooming and bonding with the herd, there was a loud backfire from the nearby road. We all startled and looked toward the noise that had broken our reverie. One of the volunteers had spontaneously put her hand over her heart.

Red was in "Sentry" mode—his entire body was on alert, and his eyes, ears, nose, and attention were targeting the direction of the frightening sound. The other horses were in alert mode, too, but they were also looking at Red.

In the back of my mind, I thought, "This could be a great moment for Marty, who is certainly watching us all."

I stepped up to Red's side and made my own body rigid and staring like his toward the threat. I blew out one, huge breath—like blowing out candles—and held my position, on alert, for a full minute. I then slouched forward, licked my lips, and blew a big sigh of relief, while turning away from the road to look at Red.

He acknowledged me with an ear flick. I stood there, licking and digging my toe into the ground. Then Red lowered his head, blew his nose, licked his lips, and placed his head behind my body.

Wow.

I had not expected that kind of compliment. By placing his head behind me, Red had said he not only trusted me, but he would let *me* be *his* Sentry. In herd dynamics, one horse is the trusted Sentry to listen to—there are some nervous horses who blow a Sentry Breath at everything, but other horses will ignore this because they know it is just a case of nerves or the "Joker" looking to get everyone in the herd riled up. Red was signaling that he trusted my Sentry opinion, which in turn allowed all the other horses to trust me as well (since he acted as their Sentry, normally). I reached over to his Friendly Button (the top of the horse's forehead is used for friendly gestures—see p. 42), and I gently stroked his head and eyes. He leaned into my hand for a few moments before moving his head away. I did a Shuddering Breath—two inhales and one, long exhale—to tell him I felt very connected to him. He blew out loudly and relaxed his lower belly in response. This said, "Me too."

All the other geldings reached back toward Rosa and the volunteers for a Check-In, touching muzzles to knuckles. They blew their noses, shook their bodies, and licked their lips.

I swished my "tail" and told the others to do the same so we could debrief about the experience before I went to talk to Marty.

All the horses swished back at us and slowly made their way back to grazing.

Having a Nice Day

"The bottom line," said Rosa, summarizing our interactions with the gelding herd, "is that we were all just having a nice day together! On a certain level, we weren't really doing much…but so much was happening at the same time! It honestly made me feel like I did back when I was a kid and could just go out in a field on my grandpa's farm and hang with the horses. It felt easy, but also so…intentional!"

We revisited the steps we had taken with the geldings. Everyone agreed that the herd had become completely at peace in those moments. Not only did these three women want those abandoned and abused horses to feel that level of wellbeing, they also acknowledged that "softening" them up this way could only make them more adoptable. It was a win-win situation.

Meeting Mr. Mist

Now that Rosa and the gang had a taste of what Horse Speak could do, I was ready to see what could be offered to poor Marty.

Even though I have worked with hundreds of horses, I never take anything for granted. Every new horse is his own being, and just because I wanted to talk to Marty did not mean he would talk to me. I always check my agenda at the door when I start on such a mission. I am not the cool kid who always wins the day. I honestly hoped (and prayed) that Marty would be open to communicating.

As we all walked back into the pasture, we noticed that Red had moved his herd off to the far right, probably to go down to the little running creek. Red lifted his head, and I nodded toward him, then looked up the hill toward Marty and swished my hand-tail toward Red. Red blew out his nose, shook his neck, and went back to eating.

Marty had come down to the edge of the tree line where there was some grass to nibble on. His body was sideways in relation to me; his head was aimed in the direction of the herd. I could see he was staring at Red, and the front of Red's head was aimed back toward him. Even though there was a good 500 feet between them, they were locked on to each other.

Interesting.

I asked the ladies to hang back and find a piece of ground where they could sit and watch. Then, I walked slowly back and forth along a parallel line to Marty's zone. I wanted to do three changes of direction while inspecting the ground so that he could see the left and right side of my body in both directions.

In Horse Speak, three changes of direction are used when determining what to do or making up your mind. Showing the side of my body meant:

1. I was not aiming head-on at him.

2. I was not afraid of him and was displaying all my body parts.

3. I was validating that *he* could do the same thing.

When I was done with this, and after tossing a few rocks toward bushes and trees for good measure, I turned to face Marty in a very "O" posture, digging my toe into the ground and loudly licking my lips. Licking only happens when a horse has relaxed enough for the soft palate to unlock. The equine soft palate is a flap of tissue that seals off the oral airway and opens up the nasal airway. This allows him to breathe through his nose but not swallow. When a horse is tense and ready to run, the palate closes so he can run safely, if necessary, without choking. A loud show of licking is a sure way to say, "Nothing to see here."

This got Marty's attention. He turned his head and neck to stare right at me, with perky ears and open nostrils. I offered a Nurturing Breath—a sound equivalent to a mother telling her baby he is safe and can suckle. In older horses, this is used to soothe another. It basically sounds like clearing your nose by sucking in and down your throat (like the noise we use to make the sound of a pig snort).

Marty nodded his head emphatically, sniffed the ground, and marched right over to me!

I was a little surprised, to say the least!

I stayed very "O" and held my knuckles out. I let Marty call the shots with the Greeting, and I did Copycat. He wanted one very soft touch, one head turn to the right, then one nostril flare touch and a look left, which he held longer and with more concern. I took initiative at this point and "blew away a bogeyman" in that direction. Marty then positioned himself behind my right shoulder to say that he was glad I could be his Sentry. By allowing me to be a Sentry for him, it was a first step in opening up to me as a Leader, a Mentor, or a Mother, because I was performing a protective role. From this 45-degree angle, I reached over for the third touch, which he let linger with very soft, inviting lips and blinking eyes.

I adjusted myself sideways to show the big gray I wanted space first, not touch. For a horse like this it is proof in the pudding that the human is not going to do the usual thing and start touching right away. Internally, of course, I wanted to just throw my arms around him and scratch his many fly bites!

I aimed my pointer finger at his Go Away Face Button, and Marty yielded his head nicely to the side and left it there. This meant that he had no intention of blundering into my space either.

I turned the front of my body away from him so that my back was to his shoulder. He reached out to my back with his Friendly Button, gently nudging me with his forehead. I turned to see his head very low, ears sideways, and an abundance of flies clearly bothering him, since no one had been able to get a fly mask on him or spray him with any sort of repellant.

Nodding my head first (to indicate movement and to ask to approach) I extended my knuckles to his withers, offering a formal invitation to Groom. He leaned into my hand and shuddered a bit. I again took initiative and reached under his neck and onto his chest. He pursed his lips as I found all the itchy spots and groaned.

Not wanting to be greedy with touch, I stopped and swished my hand-tail as I walked away. I moved my body in a sauntering motion—as though I had a good cowboy swagger—to show him there was no pressure.

Marty followed.

As I approached them, I told Rosa and the two volunteers to stand up and adopt an "O" posture. Marty and I approached them, and he made his way down the line of people, sniffing each knuckle three times before moving onto the next person. Then he walked away and circled back.

He stood with his head low, his lips drooping. His eyes were soft, and his ears were relaxed. I quietly told everyone to blink a lot, wiggle their lips, and relax their necks by making a slow "no" gesture. Marty copied this, shaking out his poll and yawning profusely. He then stretched out his back, and rocked from foot to foot. We rocked from foot to foot, too.

Marty was initiating deeper and deeper levels of relaxation throughout his body and asking to see if we could all Copycat. Now I needed to ask some questions of him.

What's Your Story?

I had everyone stand a little sideways to show connection to Marty, but no agenda. Then I approached him and went through all his Buttons using my pointer finger lightly on or just near his body. He yielded his face, neck, shoulder (which moves the front feet), and girth. When I reached for the Jump-Up Button (about 6 inches back from the Girth Button—see p. 42), I was a good foot away from it, still standing at his shoulder in case this button was a problem.

When I am gathering information about a new horse, it is essential at some point to go through all 13 Buttons in a row. Any stored anxiety or bad experiences will be revealed here, and then we can at least begin to work through them.

Can I Have the Keys?

Horses need to follow each other, but they also need to be driven forward. The driver (the horse behind) says, "You go on ahead—I've got your back and will kick a coyote if one shows up." The meekest horses stay in the middle of the herd, following a horse higher in the pecking order, and being protected from the back by another with the skills to keep his cool while driving the herd forward. Many horses fall into the "center of the herd" category, which means they do not want to lead, nor do they want to drive. Offering both roles is important.

Marty had already said I could be his Sentry, which meant he was open to *following* me. Would he also let me *drive*?

Standing up taller (broadcasting my intention to do something), I aimed my pointer finger toward his Hip-Drive Button located near the dock of the tail. I only needed to point and hold still; this is a very sensitive button and it is easily noticed. Sometimes horses are unsure about whether you want them to leave or just give you space. I did not want Marty to leave, so I tried to put only the slightest of pressure on it.

AHA MOMENT

As I aimed for Marty's Jump-Up Button, his head rose high, and his ears went back. He pulled a sour face, and I could feel him want to leave. Quickly, I retracted my hand, and stepped three steps back to take all the pressure off, like dropping a hot potato. He did not leave.

Phew.

I could see he suddenly had a faraway look in his eyes. I blinked, licked, wiggled my lips, shook my head lightly side to side, and dug my toe into the ground. Whatever "story" was stored up in that Button, it really troubled this horse. After a minute, he seemed to see me again, and he dropped his head and shook his whole body, as though snapping out of a trance.

From where I was—farther away this time—I "lightly" pointed at the same Button while in a deeper, lower "O" posture. Marty grimaced again but kept looking at me. He blew out his nose loudly and walked toward me to do a Check-In with my knuckles.

Whatever his troubling memories where, he was hanging in there with me to try and let them go.

I didn't want to linger too long on this topic, so I move my orientation around the outside of his "bubble" by taking big, slow, defined steps until I was aimed at his rump. I had stayed in "O" posture to do this, and I was a good 3 feet away.

The gray immediately raised his head, and he watched me from the corner of his eye. He had a "hard" look on his face as he tried to determine what to do. I explained my actions to Rosa and the volunteers because this maneuver can be hard to understand. All it looked like to the observer was that I was standing there, pointing at his butt, and he was standing there, looking back at me. Someone suggested I cluck or wave to make him move. I responded that this was probably the second most-misunderstood aspect of communicating with horses (the first being how to say "Hello"). We have all been taught to shoo horses into movement, and this seems so natural to most of us that it can take some "unlearning" to really get how subtle horses usually are when using their Buttons.

Horses that are friendly with each other will rub their faces or chins on each other's rumps, and they will sometimes even use their Friendly Button or Go

Away Face Button to push another horse forward or sideways. A good Leader only needs to use his hard eyes and maybe a grimace (that face horses make that looks like they sucked on a lemon) to send a whole bunch of horses moving.

Marty finally stepped over with his hind end about one foot, but his tail was tucked, and his head was high. His ears were backward in concentration and a little aggravation. As soon as he moved, I also moved away, dropping my pointing hand like a hot potato and looking down at the ground, then up at his eyes, blinking, and saying, "Thank you," out loud. This was the point where I wanted to start blending my Horse Speak body language with my typical human body language. Words elicit certain feelings, and our bodies react with micro-movements to the feelings we are having. A clear link between my voice and my micro-movements could help a horse start to gain clarity about what was "normal" human body language. Once we talk out loud, our "insides" and our "outsides" match, and this congruence helps horses "read" us better.

Marty paused for a long moment. Then he blew out a big breath and turned to face me. Nodding his head, he moved it to the side and "popped" his shoulder toward me. I had been welcomed to hang out there.

This was a very, very bright horse. He could tell already that I was trying to make him feel safe. As I approached him, I had the urge to laugh out loud, because I had the strongest sensation that he was looking at me and thinking, "Lady, you're nice and all, but you do *not* look like you could kick a coyote."

It was time to invite Rosa and the volunteers over to meet him.

The Berlin Wall

Marty had been in survival mode for so long, isolated behind a seemingly impenetrable wall of fear and disinterest, that helping him accept a group of people was important for him to be able to cross the threshold and start rejoining the group. He had already made huge efforts: he had come to me, said hello to the group, and tried to communicate about what troubled him.

The problem with walls, though, is that when we get used to having them around, their loss—even if it is for the best—is still a strange feeling.

I was going to try to help Marty by flooding him with new information and a different experience with our small group of people. If he could sustain contact with us and tolerate connection and even touch from everyone, he was going to be more likely to let that wall down for good.

Marty was a loose horse on the edge of a hillside, forest, and open pasture. There was an entire herd of geldings nearby that was taking more than a little interest in what was going on with him. There were plenty of options, in other words, if he wanted to leave. Choosing to stay with us and go through this process was a huge gift—one that I did not want to take for granted. At the same time, I felt that if I didn't push a little bit in the right way at the right time, I wasn't entirely sure Marty would be any easier to catch the next day.

I outlined my intentions to Rosa and the two volunteers, and I modeled going up to Marty, doing a Check-In with his muzzle, and then stepping to the side of him to keep the pressure off while scratching one of his many itchy spots. I held my position in scratch mode for about a minute, then stepped away from him and swished my hand-tail.

Happy Horses

Rosa lined up to go first after me. As she approached Marty, she stood a little too straight, and he put his head to the side in Go Away Face to tell her he was respectful, but he also leaned away from her. Taken together, this asked her to tone it down a notch. Deferring Space is an offer; it means the horse is giving you room. When horses give each other room, there is generally a pause—a two-way sign of respect that for us may seem like the space in which a "Thank you," would fit in a human conversation. To simply pause here and offer to do our own version of softening, like making an "O" posture, turning away, or lowering our intensity was a good idea. In the case of Marty, his Deferring Space included a significant lean away from Rosa. This signaled his willingness to leave altogether if she simply kept walking. Marty was "telling" her she could have all the room she wanted and even *more* room if she was "coming on strong." Rosa caught on to this before I could say anything and relaxed her torso, commenting that she didn't realize how "X" her body was by default.

The rest of their interaction was lovely, and her hand ventured under Marty's belly to scratch him there. He was a little nervous at first, but the pleasure of it overwhelmed his anxiety.

The first volunteer overexaggerated her "O," thinking she was trying to keep him calm. Marty dropped his nose to the ground in "Aw-Shucks" to tell her he was no threat to her. She noted then that she was now realizing that she tiptoed a bit too much around the horses that she knew had issues. With Marty she could see that this did not inspire confidence nor was it soothing—instead it made the horse feel *he* had to take care of *her*!

She also became aware as she scratched the big gray that her "O" posture kept encouraging him to bring his muzzle around to her bellybutton. She did not always remember to bring her knuckles forward for his Check-In, so at one point he nudged her tummy. I told her that Marty was telling her that if she did not give him a place to "land" then he was lost as to how to connect with her. After that she brought the knuckles of her extra hand forward as soon as she saw his head come toward her. She also practiced using his Go Away Face Button and stood a little straighter to keep her "bubble of personal space" a little clearer. This woman was finding a good balance of being soft enough to welcome him and firm enough to let him know where to be—the boundaries that are so important to horse-human relationships.

The last member of our group to approach Marty was pretty even about her "X" and "O," having watched and learned from the first two, but she scratched the horse much too quickly with an up-and-down motion—we had to find a middle ground about how to touch a horse.

I had her step away from Marty to give him some space and so I could demonstrate on her what different degrees of touch might feel like on a horse. When I scratched quickly up and down, modeling after what she had done with Marty, the volunteer crinkled her nose and frowned. "Oh my!" she said. "I had no idea. I thought they liked a firm scratch!"

As I've mentioned, up-and-down strokes or scratches go against the haircoat, and some horses really hate it. I demonstrated a circular motion that was more like massage than frantic scratching so the volunteer could feel the difference. Then, apologizing to Marty in advance, I told everyone to watch his reaction as I first offered him the comfortable, circular scratching—the gray responded by lifting his head and stretching his neck forward while tensing his upper lip. His eyes were soft, and he even groaned a little. Stepping away to signal to him I was changing something, I then returned and did the frantic up and down movement—he again lifted his head but this time pulled it backward; his ears went back, his eyes tensed, and his lips looked pursed.

Everyone watched closely, and someone wondered aloud what a "happy horse" really looked like.

Turning to look at Marty, I dropped my shoulders, flexed my neck side to side, wiggled my lips, and blinked as though I would fall down, asleep, right there at his feet. Rocking slightly on my feet, side to side, I reached out to hold his withers, and he began rocking slightly, too. The gray horse wiggled his lips, closed his eyes, and allowed his head and neck to unlock and drop forward. His shoulders seemed to stop bracing and his lower belly began deep breathing as I took long, slow breaths beside him.

I removed my hand from his withers and allowed my head and neck to drop forward toward the ground. Marty copied me, and then he closed his eyes.

We remained in this position as the horse took a short nap.

"This is the look of a 'happy horse,'" I said.

Like us, horses can get excited, and certainly excitement can be part of happiness. But, on any given day a horse is always looking for *that* level of release—true Zero—to be content.

Happy looks like Zero.

Letting Go

The only thing we really needed to "do" with Marty was to continue helping the big gelding find and keep his Zero. The most amazing thing I have learned in teaching Horse Speak is that once a horse has found or rediscovered his state of Zero, he will not only seek to keep it, he will try to help his humans go there, too.

In fact, returning to the state of Zero, and having this be the ultimate platform from which all other activities start and end, means that all the little idiosyncrasies that horses display—often termed "issues" or "vices"—start to vanish.

Instead of trying to address equine vices as though they each stand alone, it is easier to understand that horses "act out" for one reason: They are stressed, and acting out is how they are trying to cope. Pawing, cribbing, pushing, fear biting, crowding, pacing, and the list most certainly goes on—all are the result of a horse that has lost his Zero.

One by one, I have witnessed hundreds of horses let go, bit by bit, of whatever their "issue" was, as they deepen their Zero.

And Ropes

Rosa had tucked a halter into her back pocket in the hopes that if unicorns did show up that day, we could get it onto Marty.

I told Rosa to approach his muzzle three times with the halter using a "hot potato" movement to end the touch. In this way, by touching the halter, Marty could also make it go away. This worked well; he blew through his nose and shook off tension.

I then suggested that Rosa just waltz up to him as though she did it all the time and slip it on like no big deal. And…it was no big deal! He just stood there!

So next step: Taking the lead rope from my back pocket, I approached him and attached it to the bottom ring of his halter.

As soon as Marty heard that snap, his eyes widened, and he stopped breathing.

Bummer.

I immediately let out all the slack in the rope and stood facing forward near his shoulder. I figured he must have some stories to tell about lead ropes, so I wouldn't make it about the rope. I would just practice "Matching Steps" (horses follow each other by paying attention to the sound of each other's footfalls—I call this "Matching Steps"). I did not want him to focus on the lead rope and become worried, so I used my feet to draw attention to the fact that I was just asking him to follow them. Taking three firm steps forward, I then stood in place, waiting for him to catch on. He took two timid steps and froze. Stepping so I was at a 45-degree angle to his shoulder, I crossed my feet, then uncrossed them, then crossed both away from him and back to him. Crossing your feet while the horse observes you is very interesting to him. He will become fascinated with what you are doing and try to figure out if he can cross his front feet, too. I usually get the feeling horses have fun with this conversation, so I call this "Fun with Feet."

Marty wiggled his lips and crossed his front feet!

I now crossed and uncrossed my feet in an arc around the whole front of his "bubble." He watched me, then he took two more steps, both crossing and uncrossing his front feet. Changing my angle so I could see his hip, I crossed and uncrossed toward his hind end. He stepped under himself with his hind feet and turned to face me. By changing the conversation from whatever had happened to him in his past that he was reacting to when I put the lead rope on to one of "Fun with Feet," I had opened him up to the here and now. Horses can overcome fear with curiosity. I believe Mother Nature put curiosity in the horse's repertoire to make up for his having to be so on-guard all the time. I had made Marty curious, and now the benefits of him "becoming present" with me would be revealed.

Suddenly, Marty started to yawn—and yawn! Bigger and bigger, opening his mouth so wide his eyes rolled back.

Good.

The gray horse was releasing whatever it was from his past—and we'd probably never know *what*. I was happy to have a different conversation with him about matching his feet to mine.

I took up a little slack on the rope, with my palm down, and sauntered forward. He resisted the pressure a little bit, but after a few moments, the anchoring sensation I sent into the lead rope helped him settle down.

I looked at Rosa.

"Let's take him to the open stall that has an attached paddock," I suggested. "That way he is not cooped up, but he is not on the side of a mountain, either."

Rosa agreed. This would be their best shot at being able to keep spending time with Marty and to get him the care he needed. There really was no telling if he would allow anyone to come up the mountain again.

I had her take the rope and march off as though in a marching band—not fast, just intentional. He perfectly Copycatted the rhythm and timing of her feet. She marched him right out the gate and down to the stall and paddock below... the minute she turned him loose, Marty dove for the sand footing and rolled. When he rose, he stood to the back of the pen, one hind leg cocked, and dozed in the sun.

Follow Up

A few months later, I heard from Rosa. Since that day with the four of us in the mountainside pasture, Marty had made huge strides in his work with people. He had become so confident to work around—even near his Jump-Up Button—that he was now the ambassador for the farm. All groups that came through to tour the rescue or volunteer time there, like 4-Hers and Pony Clubbers, met Marty first.

Rosa had started riding him, as well, and he had returned to the trail with gusto. In fact, he was such a delight that Rosa had decided to keep him for herself. His backstory and his glorious transformation made her feel so connected to him that she just couldn't bear to send him off anywhere else.

The Long Road

The road to rehabilitation for horses in situations like Marty's can be challenging, and this was, in fact, one of the driving forces behind my effort to uncover better and better ways to connect with and communicate with horses. Unfortunately, for many horses at rescues, the good intentions of those who initially saved them from trauma or neglect are not enough to evoke a turnaround. Animals that have been through traumatic events can suffer a version of post-traumatic stress disorder (PTSD), and what's worse, the things that serve as "triggers" can be hidden. It is not uncommon for a horse to have a violent reaction to something seemingly commonplace. With Horse Speak, it is my hope that we can slow it down enough, and come to understand enough, that dangerous scenarios can be avoided on the path to rehabilitation.

LICK AND CHEW

The Greeting ritual can be used as a kind of diagnostic tool. Horses use it to size each other up, but we can use it to summarize where the horse is having problems connecting, as well as how to begin creating a new relationship with him. We also define limits and boundaries within the first moments of Greeting, and this is especially important for abused animals.

Unlike humans who suffer from PTSD, I have found that horses are much easier to "bring back." Severe cases can still take some time—even a few years—but in almost all cases there can be enough connection within the first few sessions using Horse Speak to warrant the horse's interest in trying.

In a horse's mind, they have simply arrived at a new barn. How are they supposed know they have been "rescued"? There is also the issue of time: Horses that have lived in a constant state of high alert need time to relax and get grounded in their bodies again. I have heard and dealt with many such stories over the years: At first such an animal seems "fine." His new owners may ride him for weeks, for instance, before suddenly, the horse exhibits dangerous, confusing, or even extreme behaviors. Unfortunately, what has usually happened is that the horse has made a new "map" of his current environment. He has memorized the times of feeding and established his role in the pecking order if there are other horses. Once the "outer world" is mapped out and predictable, the "inner world" rises to the surface. And, while a horse can map the outer world, he is at a loss to renegotiate his inner world on his own. He does not know how to initiate his own Zero again (the closest he may get to this is to simply demand to be left alone) nor does he know how to find Zero in people in his life. Rehabilitation needs to begin with enough rapport in the first five minutes of meeting a horse that he can begin finding his Zero *that day*.

There are certain training methods that I think are more effective for certain types of horse personalities or certain horse-human connections, but this is not cookie cutter. In the long run, horses don't really care what sort of cooking class we are into (unless they really love lobster and you insist on making shepherd's pie!) The bottom line is that any conscientious training method has both its advantages and its shortcomings; it is up to the person using it to be aware of and fill in "The Gap" when it shows up.

Horse Speak is the conversation you can maintain before, during, and after whatever kind of "work" you want to do with a horse. Most horses don't mind work, and some even thrive on it. Horse Speak offers the opportunity to comment on the process to each other, making the time we spend with our horses that much richer.

Chapter 9

Hope Heals

I taught a course in Equine-Assisted Learning (EAL) for about eight years at a college that specialized in students with learning disabilities. These students showed up for my class, bearing the burden of having grown up struggling in one way or another to learn. Some of them also suffered from anxiety, which varied in degree but in some cases involved multiple or severe panic attacks.

My goal was to give these amazing, brave souls a new experience in connection, not only with horses, but with each other…and themselves. Plus, because my attention is firmly grounded in the horse's view of the world, it was possible to create a program in which the school horses that the college leased for the semester were also enriched.

Everyone benefitted, in the end. But the beginning could sometimes be challenging.

One such beginning was particularly tough.

Expectations

We arrived at the barn around seven at night, the usual time for our class. Due to the sensitive nature of my work, coupled with the need to keep my group of students as calm as possible, I set myself up for success by running the course in the evening once everyone else at the barn had gone home, and after the horses had all had dinner.

At the beginning of each semester, I would go to the office and look at the roster of horses I could use. I piggybacked off a regular therapeutic riding program run out of the same barn, and the horses were often coming and going as needed. There might be a few horses I knew, and (more likely) there were a few I didn't. Since my program helped the horses perform better, I was often tossed the "problem" ones to "make friendly."

The first class is really just an orientation. As I introduced my students to each horse, I interpreted the horse's personality and explained how I was reading his facial cues to do it. After about the third horse, my class started getting into the game, evaluating right along with me. It was always amazing to me how easy it was to teach my students to "see" in the way you need to when looking at equine body language. So many times adults who are already set in their ways have a much harder time learning to see and interpret.

We finally arrived at the last horse—a mare that was hiding in the back of her stall. I blew out three times to invite her to come say hello to my knuckles, and she refused. She held herself very stiffly and her breathing was shallow. My class wasted no time in shouting out possible meanings for her behavior.

One girl came up close to the edge of the stall and quietly stated that the mare looked terribly unhappy. I commented that perhaps she felt connected somehow to the state this horse was in. The girl, whose name was Lianna, nodded in agreement and took a big breath. The mare cocked an ear her way and took a breath, too.

I have my students double up with horses for safety reasons (so there is always a buddy). Lianna was the first to sign up to handle this mare. The horse's name was Hope.

Because all my students in the program were over the age of 18, they were not required to tell me about their personal learning disabilities or any other issues that haunted them, as well. I didn't pry, but I always left the door open, so to speak, for them talk to me if they wanted to. Lianna confessed on the bus ride back to campus that she suffered terribly from panic attacks and that Hope had looked like "a giant panic attack" to her. I made a mental note of this and quietly began working on ways I could anchor and ground both in the effort to help them work together.

The next week, I spent a good deal of time teaching the class how to approach the horse in the stall, place the halter on, and use their breathing to stay at Zero while doing it. We would not lead horses out of their stalls until both humans and horses were at Zero. I wanted to set each student up from the get-go to be responsible for his or her horse's emotional calm.

The first thing they learned to watch for was a high, tense head. The first skills they all learned were to use breathing, grounding through their feet, and—possibly—healthy forms of touch, such as "cupping" (see p. 48) and Tellington Method T Touches, to relax the horse. It is in our nature to want to reach out and pat an animal, but as I've explained in this book, horses often do not receive this as well as we wish, nor do they find it soothing when they are tense. Of course, on the opposite side of the spectrum, I had some school horses that simply used my students as scratching posts, and with those types, I helped students set up healthy boundaries. The horses needed to be taught "good touch," as well.

This particular class was doing very well, with all finding their way toward creating and keeping Zero while opening the stall door, putting on a halter, then taking off the halter and giving their buddy a chance to try. I had everyone repeat this exercise three times, because by the third time, both the students and the horses had settled into a nice rhythm, and everyone was feeling successful and confident.

Everyone, that is, except Lianna and Hope. Lianna's buddy—a plucky girl named Shelly—had grown up with horses, and she marched right in, plunked the halter on Hope's head, and stood there petting her. While the young woman was not afraid, Shelly needed to become aware of Hope's anxiety levels. Lianna, on the other hand, was all *too* aware of the horse's issues; she could not even approach the mare due to her own anxiety rising as soon as she entered the stall.

Far from being a drawback, this was the kind of situation I was looking for. There was always at least one pairing every semester that presented interesting challenges, and this was where I could step in to provide valuable, "teachable moments."

The Teacher Becomes the Student

I asked everyone to head down the aisle to the indoor arena. The arena was set up with a barrier near the entrance so that the onlookers would have a safe place to sit and watch lessons taking place. This enabled me to turn a horse loose and demonstrate a broader spectrum of reading equine body language.

The students had all left the stalls by the time I went in to lead Hope out myself, so I was alone when she nipped me.

It was one of those moments…I knew she was upset and like a tightly wound adder, but I thought I would soothe her and ask her to come with me anyway, thinking being turned loose for a nice roll in the arena sand would do her good.

It wasn't a bad bite—in fact, her teeth just grazed my arm, so it was more like a warning. Since it was late fall, I had a fairly thick coat on. I was fine. But now my alarm bells were going off! Why was this horse in a therapeutic riding program? One makes certain assumptions about horses that are deemed "acceptable" in such programs, and mine had been that even though this mare was tense, she wasn't a danger. I gave Hope my full attention and made an "X" posture to block any further connection for the time being. Engaging my core, I held her in place in the corner of her stall, and I took a significant step away from her to give her space, as well. Dealing with aggression is one of those situations in which *any* urge to strike must be checked. Horses that have become aggressive with people have had something go terribly wrong, some-where, and the last thing I want to do was add to it.

As soon as I stepped away, she took a breath and moved her head to the side slightly in a Go Away Face offer. I moved my own head away slightly, breathing audibly. In this way, we had this exchange:

Me: "I really didn't like that."

Hope: "I really didn't like that either."

Me: "Let's think about this."

Hope: "Yes, and I will give you some room to do that."

Me: "I agree."

I took three deep breaths, and then stepped in a clear arc toward her head, looking right at her halter. Horses watch where your eyes go, much as they would watch a predator's gaze. Looking right into a horse's eyes is not only fine but good for the relationship—if you look *softly*. By stepping deliberately in an arc, I could let her know clearly what my intentions were (simply to attach the lead rope). Stopping about a foot away, I took a breath and nodded my head to ask permission to try this again.

Why ask permission? Why not simply tell her who was boss? For one reason, I was about to expose my entire class to her, so the more I could do to get her on board with me, the better my chances were of undoing whatever was making her feel so tense. Getting angry at a horse that is angry is a losing proposition. Certainly, as a trainer I can enter a "battle stance" with a horse in a pinch (if that is the only way out and my life is in danger); however, two wrongs don't make a right. I know from having dealt with hundreds of aggres-sive horses that lurking beneath what seems like nonnegotiable anger is almost always an experience where the horse felt so trapped that the only way out in his mind was to fight for his life. Fear is the motivation for almost every sort of aggression you find in a horse. The only exception may be a mother protecting her foal or a stallion defending his herd. Horses essentially live in a constant state of near-panic—any stimulus that comes along just outside of his understanding can send even a stoic horse into a flight response in about 20 seconds. Mother Nature put that there to protect their species.

Human beings are often referred to as the "hunter-gatherer" type of predator. The "gatherer" side of our nature gets along much better with horses than the "hunter" side. This can seem confusing to some because for the last few thousand years, horses were used as war machines and hunting allies. When a horse's loyalty is cultivated, he becomes bonded to his rider, and in this way will certainly protect the human the way a mare protects her young or a stallion protects his herd. Horses know it is a dangerous world; marching into battle or off to hunt is just a "day in the life."

As far as Hope was concerned, I was not intending to ride her bridle-less into battle; however, I did not want her to perceive the lead rope as a battle of wills, either.

Hurry Slowly

Hope acknowledged my head nod with a Go Away Face, licking her lips and cocking a back foot. Although her ears were concentrating backward and her face was tense, she was relaxing just enough to say that although she didn't usually like what people wanted, she would hear me out.

Excellent.

Without further ado, I put the lead rope on and moved in a steady, predictable manner out of her stall, "Matching Steps" all the way to the arena. About halfway down the aisle, Hope blew out her nose and shook her head a bit to let her stress go. Her walk became calmer and her head lowered. She reached over and gently touched my outstretched knuckles to let me know that she liked the way we were walking together. Hope was feeling the flow of my movement and becoming grounded by my predictable footfalls. By the time we reached the indoor, she was much calmer, and her eye had softened a little. As soon as we moved over the threshold, however, her tension came back, and her head lifted, ears pinned, eyes tented, and lips pinched together as though she just sucked on a lemon.

I turned her loose, and closed the gate of the indoor enclosure so she was free to move around while my students and I could watch on the other side of the barricade.

Briefly I explained that she was very "grumpy" about coming in the arena, and invited my students to begin reporting what they could observe from her body language. They eagerly offered a list of observable postures: her legs were stiff, her tail was tucked, her face was tense, and so on.

Then I asked them what they thought we could do to help her feel less stressed. Most of the students in this group had little to no real horse experience, but Shelly offered that when a horse got like that, her father always made him "run it off." Another student, Bob, stated that she was just being sour, and his grandfather would have made her work harder.

As their other classmates considered these options, Lianna asked: "But, if she is unhappy, how does that help?"

Shelly replied, "I don't know, but it seems to take the edge off."

Bob piped up, "Yeah—because if they're really tired, then they just act calmer."

I asked the group if sports or exercise helped them feel calmer. A few of the students agreed that even just going for a walk sometimes helped "get it out."

I was interested in allowing them to come to conclusions that accepted many possibilities, and it *was* possible that asking Hope to run around would help her release tension. I knew the standards at this riding school included longeing all program horses each day, either via free-schooling or on a line, and since Hope was a school horse, I knew she was accustomed to being worked that way. I decided to leave her loose in the arena while I picked up one of the less intimidating training whips leaning nearby. I was curious about what she really thought about free-longeing, and although I had my suspicions, I wanted the students to come to their own conclusions based on what they could perceive and experience. I asked the students to watch for signs of relaxation or signs of increased stress. The fact is that some horses surprise you and simply move off to "do the thing" without much fuss—you never know.

To Run or Not to Run

I greeted Hope, who strode over to Check-In with my knuckles with some eagerness, but then immediately wanted to push past me to the gate. Stepping a good 4 feet away from her, I pointed the whip toward her Go Away Face Button just to ask for room. I had no idea how she felt about free-longeing, or if she had ever been round penned, and if so if it had been done well or poorly. Just asking for a little space was a safe way to begin this conversation.

Hope turned away, and moved off. She swished her tail and pinned her ears, looking backward at me. Although she seemed to understand that we were going to have a longe session (she moved off immediately; there was no mystery about her expectation) this was done in a very defensive way. So I just stood there, not wanting to open a can of worms. The students all made note of how little I had done and how she seemed to be mad about it. In some cases, people working with horses believe that horses "need to get their bucks out" and either ignore such defensiveness or even seek it with the idea of releasing it. To me, this reaction from Hope indicated I was scratching the tip of the iceberg. I did not know yet if this horse had come to believe that her defensiveness was simply what was expected from her, or if she was authentically disagreeing with the very notion of being sent out on a schooling circle. By backing off immediately and making an "O" posture, I sent her a message, saying, "Thank you, that will do." This effectively "turned off" the conversation, alerting her to the fact that I was looking for something else and did not need or expect her to "buck it out."

The students were curious about why I backed off so soon and why the horse seemed so intense. I asked if they could relate to feeling already overwhelmed and then have "just one more thing" added that could make it all seem like too much. Everyone nodded.

I told them I didn't want to increase Hope's bad feelings, but I did want to tell her it was okay to run it off if that was what *she* actually wanted to do. Explaining this, I aimed the whip toward her Girth Button (see p. 42). This meant that even though I wanted her to move, I still wanted us to be connected.

"No, we're not!" she said and took off at a gallop.

I stayed in my spot and allowed her to run and buck on the other end of the ring. When she eventually made a beeline for me, I aimed the whip at her Go Away Face Button, and she veered off about 15 feet away from me as though she had hit an electric fence. She came to a full stop and just stared at me, wondering about it. Whether she made a beeline for me to intimidate me, or because she was nervous and seeking security, or a little of both, the answer I gave her was "give me room." By reminding her that I wanted room, too, I could begin to give her new ideas about connecting with me, and with my students.

I swished my hand down by my thigh to simulate a tail-swish "ending" and left the enclosure. My students began immediately sharing their insights.

Shelly stated that she knew her dad would have just kept pushing the mare to run it out and wondered why I stopped. I asked the group if what Hope was doing looked like exercise or like it was fun, or if it looked upset and stressed.

They could all see she was stressed. I agreed that a tired horse—or human for that matter—would behave more calmly, but I asked them what strategies they used when they were anxious about a test, for instance. Several people admitted that they suffered from generalized anxiety and worked with techniques to self-soothe in healthy ways. Some liked breathing techniques, others did meditation, and one kid simply spent as much time as possible in one of the several "quiet rooms" at the school designed to lower stress.

They all agreed that when they were anxious, they needed to focus on stress relief, which usually meant staying still. This was the same answer I was giving Hope: stay still and find your Zero.

Finding Zero

I went back in with Hope, leaving the whip outside. Taking several deep breaths, I rounded my posture into an "O" and extended my knuckles toward her. She hesitated, but then came over and stood calmly in front of me. I told the students to practice "finding Zero" with me: We all adopted an "O" posture, breathed deeply, and began to actively do a "body scan," checking in with the various parts of our bodies and releasing tension in our necks, shoulders, and arms, and then allowing that tension to go into the ground. It only took about three minutes for Hope to shake her head and neck, and drop her nose to the ground.

Then Hope took it to the next level: She carefully nosed toward my boot while her head was still almost to the ground, which was a way to let me know she wanted me to move away, although she was being respectful about it. I took one step back, which was a reply that said simply, "Okay."

Hope raised her head to shoulder level, which said that she was keeping her cool, and flopped her ears sideways to say she was feeling better. She walked off slowly and carefully, making one complete circle in front of us, and ending with her gaze back upon us. When a horse moves away carefully and shows you all his sides, he is sharing himself more deeply with you: "Here is all of me, I am ready to talk with you." Sometimes this happens as Hope did it, walking a circle; sometimes the horse stops and presents certain Buttons, lingering on one or another area to indicate what he thinks we should talk about. For instance, if a horse moves away slowly and carefully, and offers his Hip-Drive Button toward you, he is saying, "We should talk about who is driving. Are you up for being responsible, or not?" I have often seen a horse do this when his owner is having a hard time emotionally. The horse may offer his rump toward someone who is not feeling strong not so much as a query ("Can you be my Leader and drive me?") but more as a statement ("You're not feeling well, are you? You don't feel up to driving to me"). I have observed needy horses swinging the rump toward a Leader, asking to be driven (which gives a great deal of comfort), and I have observed stoic horses put a Bully in his place by turning the rump to him, in effect yelling, "You are *not* fit to drive!"

Horse Speak is a nuanced form of communication. Topics of discussion between horses may be pragmatic and practical, but their ability to comment on feelings is of utmost importance. In fact, the feelings of the herd determine the safety and security within that group. This is why horses can be so "healing" to be around: Feelings are the basis of what they are interested in talking about.

The class was intrigued by what Hope seemed to be saying. They sensed that she was ready to be present with us on a different level. I had each one come to the edge of the arena and extend a fist, knuckles up. I still wanted to keep some distance between my group and Hope, so I put the lead rope on her to guide her through Greeting all 15 students.

At first, Hope seemed a little overwhelmed. She wanted to circle away after only Greeting two people. We all paused for a few moments, and everyone went back to deep breathing. I told the students to try a version of Greeting that is speedier: a simple 1-2-3 touch on her nose with a long out breath on number three.

This worked much better for Hope. She was interested in the faster sequence of touches and flared her nostrils in time with the 1-2-3 bumps from my students. When she reached Lianna, however, something changed. Hope flared her nostrils and delicately touched Lianna's knuckles three times, then three more, then three more, for three sets. This increase in delicate touching and nostril flare meant that the relationship between the two was more complex, and they needed time to sort things out.

AHA MOMENT

As they lingered with each other, I saw a change come over both Hope and Lianna. There seemed to be some sort of natural connection and understanding between them. Lianna spoke to it, saying, "I feel something when I am with this horse, but I don't know what it is."

I told her to sit with it a while and see if she got some clarity. Hope went on to Greet the rest of the class, and when she was done, I turned her loose one more time. She moved away a few feet and had a good roll in the sand, which delighted us all.

After I put Hope away, the class reassembled, and we talked about some of the topics that being with Hope had brought to the fore: tough feelings like anger and anxiety. I told them it would be great for Hope to be able to free longe to work out some of her stress, as long as it felt good to her, and didn't add *more* stress. As our class progressed, we would invite Hope to relate to longeing in a more useful way: We would practice finding and keeping our Zero, which would help her find and keep her own.

Snow

A few weeks went by, and Lianna and Hope were making real progress with each other. Groundwork lessons encouraged all the students and horses to stretch their comfort zones a little bit more each week but always focused on keeping both human and horse at Zero on the inside. If either one got too edgy, the students were responsible for sensing this, stopping what they were doing, and attending to the needs of the moment. This meant that some classes had students and horses off to the side for most of each session as they practiced finding and keeping their Zero.

One evening toward the end of the semester, it had been snowing, and the pitched roof of the indoor was quite laden. We were just beginning to work and everyone had spread out around the arena when a big hunk of snow suddenly fell from the roof to the ground outside. The noise was deafening, and everyone jumped. Lianna dropped the lead rope when Hope spooked, doubling over as she fought the onset of a panic attack. I immediately made my way toward her, but it was Hope that got there first, coming back, arching her neck, and gently laying her head and neck over the girl.

I stopped and watched as Lianna looked up to see how Hope was draping over her. For a moment, the girl was even more nervous and scooted out from under the mare's neck, but two or three students called out, "She's helping you! It's ok!" Lianna looked toward me, looking for guidance, wondering if what her classmates were saying was true.

"It's true…you can let her help you," I reassured her, "or just step away if it's too uncomfortable."

Lianna turned and looked into Hope's eyes, and then spontaneously wrapped her arms around the mare's neck. Hope remained still, pulling the young woman closer to her by pressing her face against Lianna's back. The pair remained in their embrace for a few minutes, then unwound and regained their composure. Lianna picked up the dangling lead rope, nervously laughing while wiping the tears and looking around. I told all the students to go ahead and hug their horses if they felt like it.

All my students were realizing that "going to Zero" was not just an annoying sidebar to getting things done every week. Several noted that it was this that had set up Lianna and Hope to connect as they just had, and that it had also prepared the rest of the class to be able to "roll with it" when the snow had fallen from the roof. My students who battled anxiety acknowledged they were able to come back to a calm place much sooner than they had in the past, and a few stated that they hadn't even been scared by the sudden noise.

A New Path

When the semester was over, Lianna confided in me that when she went back to her grandfather's ranch, she would have an entirely new way to relate to horses. This, she said, had been one of her secret goals.

As it turned out, Lianna stayed in touch with me through the years, and ended up volunteering at a local therapeutic riding center, and later going back to school for it. Ultimately, she became a farrier, using her Horse Speak skills to help her four-legged clients relax. Lianna had thought she was getting help for her severe anxiety when she joined my class, but it turned out she found her life's path, as well.

Hope was sold not long after the semester ended to a woman who wanted a safe horse to use on the trail. The mare never really enjoyed carrying many different people all day, but she did enjoy a singular relationship. About a year later, her new owner came by the barn to give us an update on Hope's progress and thank us for selling her the mare. I asked if Hope ever offered to hug her. The woman looked surprised for a moment, then admitted, "Well, yes! You know about that? I thought I was imagining it, but she will press her face into my body and sort of scoop me in toward her every now and then."

I told her the story of Hope and Lianna, and how much it had impacted that whole group of students. I said to sniff Hope's neck as a reply, as that is how horses tell each other they're connected.

She was very eager to run right home and do just that.

LICK AND CHEW

The bond between the tense mare Hope and anxious student Lianna was only possible because their connection was based on Lianna's compassion for Hope's frustration, struggle, and need for Zero. Once Lianna and Hope began to work toward Zero in everything they did together, they both experienced immediate and long-term benefits. Rather than focusing on Hope's obedience only, or Lianna's anxiety only, as though those elements stood alone, the integrity of the relationship was the focus. When Lianna brought enough Zero to Hope, the mare easily reciprocated. The lasting effect caused them both to be able to reach deeper, and find a way beyond their previous inhibitions. And, the mutual respect and compassion they nurtured in each other went past their immediate relationship, finding its way into the rest of their lives.

Chapter 10

The Journey Home

Ann had once enjoyed the good fortune of living in a cottage with a barn on a 100-acre property. She had owned a very special horse named Royal, and since she worked as a yoga instructor from her home, she was able to spend most of her spare time just "being" with her horse. It was the type of arrangement where Royal didn't need to be locked up…and he sometimes stuck his nose in an open window if he was bored and wanted to see what she was doing. For many horse lovers, this scenario sounds like a dream come true. It certainly was for Ann!

After several years together, Royal became ill. He put up a good fight, but eventually passed away. Devastated, Ann left the cottage with the barn, got married, and moved to the city.

After a few years, however, her passion for horses overcame her sorrow. And one day she came across an advertisement for a reasonably priced horse—that looked just like her Royal.

Ann didn't hesitate, immediately arranging to meet the horse—an off-the-track Thoroughbred named Journey. Much to the surprise of his current owners, Ann and Journey seemed to get along right away. She was sold. Wasting no time, she moved this new horse to her mother's small farm a few hours away from her home in the city. She envisioned going to the farm on weekends and riding the endless trails.

Only a few weeks later, however, she started to have her suspicions as to why this horse had been so reasonably priced, and why his owners had been so surprised when they had gotten along. As Journey settled into his new home, a "mean side" started to show up. For reasons Ann could not fathom, he would suddenly glaze over, and rear, kick, or bite.

At first Ann applied herself to trying to figure out what the triggers were, but as time went on, she came to realize that she simply could not figure out her horse, no matter how hard she tried. Things degenerated to the point where she could not even go near him without a whip in her hand for self-defense. Finally, even that failed: One day Journey grabbed her by the upper arm, nearly breaking it as he tossed her like a rag doll several feet away.

Ann began searching for a trainer or teacher who could help her—one who wouldn't beat her horse or blame her. After a year of disappointing experiences, she was about ready to give up completely. She reached out to me in a state of desperation.

I was traveling to her area for a clinic and said I would carve out some time to meet with her and see what could be done. We made arrangements for me to go to where Journey was stabled. I did not want such a horse being trailered to a clinic, where he might put himself and others at risk.

Starting Over

By the time I met Journey, Ann had done some homework and tracked down what she could of his history. He had raced until he was four, and then, considered washed up, he'd been gelded and sold off at auction. Since then, he had been through several homes, and each time trainers had been called in to try and help solve his issues. Through it all he only seemed to get worse.

Now that he was 11, Ann felt for certain that she was Journey's last hope. And if she could not help him, she would not sell him either, because she felt he was a danger to anyone. She had decided he could live out his days on the farm, and no one would touch him. But for her, this added salt to the wound of missing her beloved Royal. Having once felt so connected and at peace with a horse, this level of disconnect and aggression was confounding to her.

Journey lived in a one-acre paddock attached to a stall, which he could go in and out of at will. There was an ancient Mustang with him, and they seemed joined at the hip.

I blew a soft greeting at the Mustang first, nodding my head and walking up and down the fence line in three changes of direction to show my interest in talking. The Mustang stared for a moment, then did an "Aw-Shucks" and breathed back at me. He took a step forward, but Journey pinned his ears and blocked his movement. The Mustang breathed toward me, then turned and walked away.

I wanted to talk to the elder horse first, thinking that this would help me introduce myself to Journey. The fact that the conversation was so rudely blocked was not a great sign…but it did give me a lot to think about. Information gathering is as important as anything else.

I changed my tactics and kicked the fence posts a little, then checked the water tub in the corner and tossed some hay into the hay bucket. I wanted to show Journey that I was a person who meant business. If I lingered on just trying to make contact with him, he would not be interested. By blocking the Mustang, he had already told me he didn't like people. He probably had a story in his head that told him I was just another trainer out to get him.

I turned my back to the horses and began talking to Ann. As we talked, I moved her to the left a step, then reached out and moved her back to the right. Whether Journey "liked" her or not, he perceived Ann as "his," and by moving her around a little bit, I was claiming her as "mine" in that moment—very similarly to how he had claimed the Mustang a few minutes before.

That got his interest. Just because he was sometimes mean to her didn't mean he didn't think she was his.

The Thoroughbred blew out his nose loudly and nodded his head deliberately. I perceived this as rather like a stallion challenging another stallion. It was possible that the later-in-life gelding had left him a bit more "studdy" than we would have liked.

Healthy stallion leadership in a balanced herd is often very tender and soft toward herd mares and foals. Stallions can and do use force to protect their herd and sometimes can be more forceful toward members of their band if they are stressed or trying to drive everyone forward in times of danger. In domestic situations, however, stallions rarely have healthy relationships with their family groups and are kept isolated instead. In many cases, the humans who own stallions want to channel all that power into a performance, but without a healthy family group to experience life with, stallions can often get out of control.

I observed Journey's overreactions to *everything*. I had no proof yet that this was the case with him, but the more I watched him, the more he reminded me of the troubled stallions I had worked with over the years. I decided to proceed with an awareness that he might be poorly socialized to begin with and possibly very unclear about healthy boundaries, even with other horses.

After a few more minutes of us ignoring him, Journey marched over to the fence. Ann was glad to see him come toward us because, she said, he could often be very reclusive. I, too, was glad to see him come over, but I also took note of the fact that he approached very high-headed, with his poll arched—more dominant communication.

I offered my knuckles to him but remained slightly out of reach. He would have to stretch his neck all the way out to say hello. As he did, he pinned his ears and rolled his eyes, acting like he would bite. I knew I was just slightly out of reach, so I did not flinch, but remained still, breathing deeply. He pulled his head away and regrouped. I turned to the side and "scanned the horizon" (looking far and wide for any threats or danger) for a half-second, then firmly stuck my fist toward him again.

This time, Journey paused for a moment and actually seemed to look at me, instead of just reacting to my presence. He reached toward my knuckle again and this time sniffed it from an inch away. As he retracted his head, I turned to the side again, and scuffed the ground in an "Aw-Shucks."

My goal was to model a formal Greeting, and to communicate I wanted him to "turn the volume down." I had told him I was aware of the environment and that I had a certain relationship with his human. I did not want to diminish him in any way, but I did aim to offer a calm leadership—the way an older mare would.

Mares, Geldings, and Stallions, Oh My!

I have been lucky enough to watch older mares teach overzealous geldings or young studs about manners. They are very serious about making the boys follow the rules of engagement, and although they can and will use their powerful hindquarters to make a statement if they have to, these mares usually simply repeat the essay on manners over and over again, drilling the adolescent behavior right out of the offenders. The "boys" are not allowed to remain close to a mare unless they are calm. In other cases, I have watched very skilled mature geldings settle uppity youngsters, but usually geldings have a little more give and take and are more relaxed, as could be seen in the case of the Mustang and Journey.

I would have to take on the manners of a mature mare to change the Thoroughbred's attitude, because it appeared having a "Whatever, dude" attitude like the Mustang was going to go nowhere.

I guessed that many previous trainers had probably taken the stance of trying to get Journey to cower in submission. That would be like a stallion taking on a stallion; I had no interest in that sort of activity or relationship.

I was going to adopt the curt, punctual dialogue of a no-nonsense teacher who has taught school for a million years and expected to get through the lesson no matter what "Little Timmy" was doing. I would not be dragged into drama by this horse. Instead I would model the code of behavior I expected him to follow. I set myself up mentally to sit right in the center of his hurricane and not budge.

Journey stared at me as I did an "Aw-Shucks" and breathed out a little. I offered my knuckles again—still at a distance—and he hesitated. Reaching out for my knuckles this third time, he kept his ears forward, looked me right in the eyes, and gently touched the edge of my hand for a second. As he moved his head away, I aimed my pointer finger at his Go Away Face Button on the side of his cheek. He stared at me in seeming disbelief, then tilted his head slightly.

Saying, "Thank you," out loud, I stepped to the side and turned my back to Journey to talk to Ann again. I wanted him to soak up what had just happened. Ann asked about my pointer finger—in this case, I had simply pointed at him, then held it up in the air like an irate teacher saying, "CLASS!" In this case, I was not going to be able to get up close to his cheek to ask him to move his face politely away—the risk of him overreacting and trying to bite was too high. I do not want to allow a horse a chance to practice bad manners, so I try not to set them up for failure.

In a situation like Journey's, where the horse did not have good social skills, I was going to have to fill in where his mother left off. I was going to have to help him remember the proper rules of engagement in his own language before I could ever hope to get him to start finding his Zero again.

"X" and "O" Together

As you've learned, there are two basic postures that contain many meanings. The "X" is meant to ask for movement or just a little space. The "O" is meant to welcome or create harmony. Talking to Journey effectively meant I had to calibrate my "X" and "O" at the same time. I wanted enough "O" to ask him to talk to me, but I had to keep enough "X" to stand my ground and keep him out of my "bubble of personal space."

Often horses that are worked at a young age, like Journey, learn that they cannot get away from people *ever*. Their space feels invaded all the time, and either they completely shut down, or they start to drive people away forcefully to preserve their own "bubble." Those attitudes can become habits, and even when the story has changed, the horse remains distant or defensive.

I suspected that this was part of Journey's problem, so my first step was to teach him that he could always ask for space and receive it—but he should do so politely and calmly. By telling *him* to give *me* space right away, then giving him space right back as a reward, I was setting the stage. I would have to model a polite request if I wanted him to know what I was looking for.

Journey made a game out of touching my hand and moving his face away, several times in a row. Each time he became softer. Finally, he walked away for a bit; I swished my "hand-tail" as he left to agree that this was a good idea. He swished, too.

Ann and I went to the house briefly, and when we returned, Journey was waiting for us at the fence. Ann was thrilled that he was so interested, and she commented that his overall demeanor looked softer. I agreed that it did, but I knew we were about to have another sort of conversation—one that Journey would absolutely need clarity about, especially if he had been dominated by trainers in the past. This conversation was about the use of assertiveness. I needed to show him I could be a strong "X"—I call it a "Level Four" intensity (Levels One, Two, and Three being the "intention," "asking," and "telling" levels of intensity—see p. 103). A proper Level Four is done between horses in the blink of an eye. Sometimes they actually bite or kick. Sometimes they miss on purpose, but the message gets across.

However, a Level Four between horses is over as soon as it's over. This is the hard part for people!

Horses being assertive know how to calibrate intensity. Humans tend to slip into aggression and get stuck there.

I have spent years learning to be *assertive* and not *aggressive*, which means that Zero is on the inside no matter what I am doing on the outside. If my insides get upset and emotional (angry, frustrated, or scared) it won't work. Because this is so important, I have a strategy that helps the human stay cool as a cucumber but creates a Level Four outward intensity that the horse absolutely believes. I save this for occasions such as

Journey presented, because misusing the strategy would ruin an ordinary conversation.

There was no way I could impart everything I knew to Ann in an hour, and I would not be back to see her and Journey's progress for a few months. I had to leave her and her horse in a better place, capable of continuing his rehabilitation while keeping her safe.

The Secret Power of a Shopping Bag

While inside the house, I asked Ann for an ordinary plastic shopping bag. Back in the barn, I grabbed a short riding crop and tied the bag to the end of it. I punched a hole in the bottom of the bag so it would not fill up with air when it moved around.

As I approached Journey, I held the crop-and-bag behind my back so I did not alarm him. He reached over the fence for a Check-In, and I breathed softly toward him. Then I stepped back one step, stood up tall, and moved the bag carefully to the front of my body. That was it. I just held it down by my feet and did not move it.

Journey reacted like a wolf had showed up, blowing and snorting toward the bag. I stepped aside, and move the crop-and-bag behind my back in one motion. Dropping it to the ground, I stepped in with a big "O" to do a Check-In with him. He wanted to linger a bit with his lips on the back of my knuckles. I allowed this, breathing deeply, then I adopted a strong "X" and pointed in the air at his Go Away Face Button, along with his Mid-Neck Button, to ask him for even more room (see p. 42). He complied nicely and quickly.

I stepped back and picked up the crop-and-bag again. Holding it low, by my feet, I pointed it toward one of his front hooves from about 5 feet away. He stepped backward as though the bag was about to eat him.

Quickly, I dropped the bag and moved in to do a Check-In again. Journey eagerly met me for the Check-In, then he stepped back and did an "Aw-Shucks," dropping his nose to the ground and blowing out. He was asking for me to keep the pressure down. I did my version of "Aw-Shucks," and walked away, leaving the bag out of it.

All I was really doing in this situation was adding believability to my "X." Journey had severely bitten Ann (and who knew how many other people); when I was no longer there, I wanted her nervous system to believe in "the power of the bag," and for Journey to know that "power" was only *assertive*—never aggressive.

As much as I wanted the Thoroughbred to come as close to me as he could while I still remained on the safe side of the fence, and as much as I wanted to develop his interest in bonding using my "O," I had to make sure the boundaries were strong. Boundaries make bonding happen—remember how I likened them to a bowl without cracks back on page 105? The bowl is the container that healthy boundaries make, and the soup the bowl holds is the nourishment of a healthy bond. Relationships need both. Journey needed the support of the fence line to know he could get away from us if he needed to—that is, I did not want him to feel he had to drive us away. And we needed it to be able to remain at Zero.

Now that Journey was keenly aware of—but not afraid—and very much engaged in this conversation, it was a good time to have Ann do her first formal Greeting with him.

Your Turn

Approaching the paddock fence, Ann held the crop-and-bag behind her back, and even just the act of doing this made her more comfortable. She was able to reach toward her horse three times and Greet him, then point to his Go Away Face Button and ask for space. He complied to each thing and appeared to become more thoughtful.

Journey was nowhere near Zero, but at least the two had a new platform to work from.

Ann practiced her "Xs" and "Os," and he practiced coming toward her and moving away. As her excitement built, Ann forgot herself and lingered too long inside the horse's "bubble of personal space," keeping her knuckles extended toward his muzzle for far too long, hoping for more affection. Like a swiftly moving storm, Journey's ears went back and his eyes rolled. He pulled his head high and backward in a "cobra" motion—like that of a snake about to strike. I quickly stepped into Ann's space with precision and drove the horse backward with my pointer finger and a little snap of my fingers at the same time. Grasping her by the shoulders, I moved Ann away from his head to be safe, but he had yielded his head away the moment I snapped my fingers.

The lesson was not lost on her.

AHA MOMENT

Suddenly, Ann had crystal-clear insight about what was happening: She missed her dear horse Royal so much that the faintest glimmer of connection with Journey caused her to override what was actually happening and no longer pay attention to the fact that he had no idea how to share affection with her yet. In her yearning for a breakthrough, she'd forgotten completely about their "bubbles of personal space," the plastic bag she had to help her be assertive, or the point of establishing healthy boundaries.

Ann realized that she needed to practice boundaries and bonding with an "easy" horse first. Her own internal struggle over wanting a deep relationship again with a horse was creating incongruity and manifesting as difficulty and hard times with Journey.

Good Ol' Coby

There was another horse on the farm: a kind, easygoing soul that Ann's mother used for riding lessons. His name was Coby.

We took a break from Journey to go visit Coby. Ann sailed through the Greeting ritual with him, and he offered a lovely Go Away Face, as well as a willingness to react to his other Buttons, which provided helpful lessons for Ann. This horse stopped on a dime the moment you looked remotely like an "X."

Coby was overjoyed to talk Horse Speak with us and was very fluent in human body language mistakes. He even began correcting Ann's bellybutton angles (she tended to leave her bellybutton toward him rather than turning it aside). Coby constantly encouraged her to stand shoulder to shoulder with him to sort out both her boundaries and her offerings to bond. He allowed some lovely contact but wasn't afraid to comment if Ann touched him mindlessly, or made the mistake of scratching him in an up-and-down manner. Coby was very kind about the whole thing, lifting his head and making a sour face when he did not like something, and rewarding her with a very low head, soft facial expression, and even licking the back of her hand when she got it right.

Suddenly, it became very clear to Ann that although she had lived with Royal and they had sorted out how to get along, she was not totally clear about how to talk to horses, in general. The more she practiced Horse Speak with Coby, the more Zero he became until finally he just took a nap.

By the time I left that day, Ann had successfully used the influence of the plastic bag to keep a better boundary between herself and Journey, and she had recreated reasonable bonding moments several times, as well. When we were done, Journey took a nap, and the old Mustang was finally able to come to the fence and say hello to us.

Keep It Rollin'

Ann's homework was to keep working with Coby to hone her Horse Speak skills and to practice boundaries and bonding with Journey *over the fence* until she felt safer about going inside the paddock with him. This process would take time, but I felt confident that between Coby's teaching and Ann's new awareness of what both her and Journey's needs actually were, they could make some progress.

A few months later I went back to see how they were progressing. Journey could stay present and follow instructions without acting out for longer and longer durations. If he did hit his "limit" he could now ask for space by yielding his head away and leaving it there, avoiding all contact. This was *much* better than feeling like he had to drive people away when he was overtaxed. In this way, he was cultivating a kind of "work ethic" that would serve them both in the years to come.

Ann had figured out what sort of affection Journey enjoyed (mostly scratching his belly). He had not bitten her again. There were occasional moments when he still resorted to making a very ugly face, but Ann would simply pull the crop-and-bag out of her back pocket, and wiggle it toward him. Having an easy way to do a Level Four intensity "X" meant she did not panic when Journey was too intense, and it was a clear way for Journey to understand he needed to back off. He would step aside, and she would, too. Sometimes they would end for a bit and try again later.

This visit we played with liberty work, which helped them both "Go Somewhere" together and learn more and more about each other in doing so. I set up barrels, cones, and ground poles, so there were many things to negotiate and talk about besides each other and how they were feeling. It is essential when rehabilitating a horse to have achievable goals to work toward, and horses enjoy manipulating objects. I told Ann to work with Journey at liberty for a week or so, and then use a long lead rope to go through some of the same obstacles. I wanted to remove any tension he might feel about being "trapped."

Progress Report

A few weeks later, I heard again from Ann. Work had progressed rapidly. The first day she used a lead rope, she noticed Journey became really concerned. She had not realized before how trapped he actually felt when he was on one. Using her newly developed skills, Ann helped Journey find his Zero on the rope and kept her Zero even when he seemed to get very high-headed. She said by the third time they worked on a lead rope, he was calm and responsive.

Ann was a wonderful yoga instructor; I had suggested that she practice some yoga around or near her horse to see what this did for him. She had begun doing it in the aisle of the barn, and Journey watched her very closely over the stall door. It wasn't long before he seemed to adjust himself and how he was standing every time she did! At one point, as Ann reached gently into a deeper form, Journey lifted his hind leg and scratched beneath it with his nose. Ann felt confident enough to enter Journey's stall to do some of her favorite yoga asanas. The Thoroughbred carefully nuzzled her with his nose. He was extremely mindful, only touching her enough to maintain contact but not to unbalance her. He seemed to want to join in somehow.

After a few more minutes of enjoying their space together, Journey retreated to his side of the stall, cocked a hip, and seemed to drift off. Ann stepped out of the stall. Her sense of the encounter was that Journey had entered into a deeper state of connection with her, and then had had enough. She was not disappointed at all: being a yoga teacher, she was familiar with how powerful it could be in redirecting a student and helping one into a deeper relationship within oneself. Ann felt it would not surprise her if Journey was experiencing some level of this.

The encounter had also helped Ann see Journey in a new light—a more familiar one. If he had been "used" as a racehorse, then his body was not his own for the first few years of his life. Thinking of him from her yoga-teacher perspective gave her new insights and compassion for helping him to develop a different association within himself, and also with her and the world in general. As a teacher, she was much more up to the challenge of his rehabilitation.

Accessing skills she already had gave her a sense of renewal when thinking about working with her horse.

Back in the Saddle

It wasn't long before I received an excited email from Ann. One day, when she had saddled and ridden Coby, Journey had come to the fence and watched. On a whim, she placed the saddle and bitless bridle on the round pen fence for Journey to explore. He sauntered over to the items, and tugged at them a little bit. She felt confident that he was interested in trying it out, so Ann saddled Journey without tying him. She added the bridle, and with all going well, Ann sat on her horse for a moment. When she asked Journey to walk off a little, he moved carefully and thoughtfully. It was a nice moment for them both—and Ann ended right there, before either of them could become tense.

After she got off, he rolled and rolled in the dirt of his paddock and took a nap.

I was thrilled to hear these two were finding their way to a better place together. I reminded Ann to keep going *slowly*—not to get greedy and expect that things with Journey were now always okay. To bring a horse back to Zero under saddle is a whole different thing than doing it on the ground. However, they were well on their way!

The fact that Ann and Journey had come this far in only a few months was actually quite impressive and a testimony to her ability to be authentic with herself and the process. Some horses take even longer than this, but to me, these horses are worth the wait. When it all comes around, there is an immense wealth of experience and trust that is worth every second.

Becoming the still-point in the center of the hurricane means you can stay true to yourself, and your horse will trust your authenticity.

Don't Freak Out

As I mentioned in the last chapter, I often see well-intentioned people "shoo-ing" a horse backward and away from a gate or stall door. The horse is high-headed and tense, and the human is usually wearing an intense scowl. The person feels she "has to" look and act like that to get the horse to give her space. Essentially, this means her "X" is not believable otherwise. But this is such a hard state to live in! No one really wants to have an adversarial relationship with a horse in which you have to flail around in order to get some simple space needs met.

The reason I begin all meetings whenever possible with the Horse Speak formal Greeting over a fence or stall door is because it is a formula for creating rapport and boundaries *at the same time*.

If you are clear and precise about using the Go Away Face Button, asking for a respectful amount of space becomes very easy. However, if you are muddying the waters by secretly feeling bad about asking for space; if you are using the wrong sort of touch (as in pressing the palm of your hand to the cheek, which actually means "bring your face to me"); if you are using your pointer finger too abruptly ("stabbing" angrily at the horse's face) or touching the wrong spot completely and using the Play Button (alongside the horse's mouth—see p. 42) instead, then negotiating space can be an ongoing struggle.

Snapping your fingers and pointing in the air toward the Go Away Face Button helps ensure people are clear about being precise in their movements and intention, as well as instilling in them the fact that horses do this all the time! Horses constantly ask each other to move their head—that way they can walk past, reach for food or water, or make other adjustments without having to also move their feet. Horses are masters at "low-calorie conversations" and when you understand their subtlety, then you can tap a vast resource of powerful communicative tools that create a deep well of trust and respect on both sides.

If a normal amount of "X" has no effect, then a plastic bag, tied to the end of a crop, can help emphasize your Level Four intensity. However, this does *not* mean you should flail around with a plastic bag and send your horse into a panic. A person can corner a horse in a round pen or paddock, or on a lead rope, and bully him into total submission, but this is not a Level Four experience of "X" that a healthy horse would *ever* use with another horse. Horses that are Bullies become that way because normal socialization with a healthy herd was stunted somewhere along the line. They have lost their Zero with other horses.

Basically, with an overreactive horse, you have to have a healthy ability to be assertive at a Level Four but *not* slide into aggressive tactics. Your Zero is believable when your Level Four "X" is believable. Just as Zero does not mean "pushover" or "doormat," Level Four does not mean "freaking out."

Meek or "mousey" energy is not a healthy Zero, and we can sense this with another human because it feels like the person just disappears; there is no one to connect to. However, aggressively shoving anyone around, human or horse, belies insecurity and fear. Being a marshmallow looks undesirable; losing your cool looks weak.

In comparison, a healthy Level Four looks safe to a horse the way an ER doctor looks trustworthy when she shows up and calmly looks at your broken leg; perhaps she even smiles at you or pats your arm reassuringly. She is certainly in charge, with a "can do" attitude that makes you feel like you can let go and trust that your leg will get fixed. However, if the doctor showed up and couldn't look you in the eye, acted shy and mumbled, or was too gruff and yelled at you, then you would doubt her ability to care for you.

Learn to be welcoming, but value yourself by valuing your personal space in your relationship with your horse.

And learn to resist drama. The temptation to rise to a horse's dysfunctional level of aggression with your own aggression is not going to offer lasting value. Certainly, in a moment of danger, one has to protect oneself. Never allow a horse to bite or kick because you don't want to be "mean." But this state is not conducive to long-term healthy relating. *It feels bad.* It plain old rots to have to live on guard around a horse or to have a horse that can never find quiet peace of mind.

When I have to use a large physical Level Four intensity to make a point with a horse that is totally out of control, I make a mental note of that, and decide right then and there the tone and pitch I want to *usually* live at in this relationship. I begin to model the more appropriate level of connection from that moment on, and if the horse tests me at some point (and horses always do) I refuse to be roused to the previous level of intensity. This is one of the reasons I prefer to have plenty of freedom for both the horse and myself by keeping a barrier between us for the first meeting (a fence, a stall door) to clear up any confusion that may be lurking for the horse. I have watched Mentor horses model the same clarity and consistency with clueless charges assigned to them, even when there is a fence between them. These healers rise to an intense level once, maybe twice. After that, they work to show the way for the underling to arrive at a better position in life with quiet determination and a level of focus and presence that would put a Tibetan monk to the test.

LICK AND CHEW

Being a teacher in your relationship with your horse makes you a good Leader. There is a difference between *training* and *teaching*. I can *train* someone about the use of a fishing rod and bait. However, *teaching* someone to fish takes patience and practice—and is also where the real value in fishing shows up.

Teaching a horse about my "bubble of personal space," and also what I like and don't like, means I am simultaneously opening the door for *him* to tell *me* his own particulars—and that is where the real value of connection shows up. In many OTTB cases, their early handling was very rigid. When I was a student, I often noted how young Thoroughbreds were commonly led with a chain slipped from the cheek ring of the halter through the lower ring and over the horse's upper gums. I have no idea why this seems to have become standard practice, but I have met many OTTBs that have real issues with their personal space and especially their face. These horses need to know they can have all the room they need to find their Zero, and it starts with the "bubble of personal space."

In the case of an "angry" or aggressive horse, establishing myself as the eye of the hurricane means I will not be drawn out into his drama. Instead I will hold my own state of Zero and invite him to find his own. When a horse has lost his Zero to the point of acting out, then the only way through is to weather the storm together. If you can maintain the calm center of the hurricane consistently enough, the horse will find his way home… to his Zero. Ann was able to find her own calm center—her Zero—and Journey was finally able to come home.

Chapter 11

When Horses Talk Back

Lisa owned a very talented 10-year-old dressage horse that gave her nothing but trouble on the ground. Her dressage instructor was very good, and together they had devised many ways of quieting Brandy's behavior, yet he had a way of spooking at the most awkward moments—in fact, his spooking was legendary. At least once every few weeks Lisa found herself struggling just to get him into the ring.

She owned four other lovely horses that roamed around her wide-open property. Some were seasoned trail horses while others were completely retired and simply enjoyed the rambling fields. Brandy was often the only reason for any of them to move faster than a casual walk. He bossed the other horses around every chance he could, and finally, Lisa had to move her two older mares to a separate paddock to avoid his constant harassment.

Lisa had attended a few of my clinics and asked me to come meet her horse to see if I could make sense of his antics. She was especially frustrated because she had owned him since he was a weanling and had done "everything right" as far as his education and training. Neither she nor her dressage instructor could figure out *why* he was so overreactive.

The Boy Who Cried Wolf

When I first arrived, I noticed the stunning blood bay horse out in the middle of a large field. He noticed me, as well, shooting his head straight up and blowing Sentry Breath at my arrival. The two geldings grazing nearby didn't even acknowledge his gesture.

Oh, boy.

This told me a great deal about Brandy's character. The other horses had declared that he was a terrible Sentry, much like "the boy who cried wolf."

Meanwhile, poor Brandy was so hypervigilant that any change in his world sent him into a panic.

Quickly, I answered him from my car, blowing a huge, sharp Sentry Breath and getting onto my tippy toes to make myself look extra alert. Fight fire with fire. The bay stared at me as though I was an alien, then he lowered his head to the ground, and lifted it back up again rapidly. This was an attempt to say, "No kidding? You know that?"

I then released a long, relaxing breath, licked my lips, and turned away from him to say that not only was I onto his game, but I did not want to be panicky around him. I would now ignore him and check out the grounds.

Lisa was walking toward my car to greet me and had paused while I performed this interaction. She was aware enough to know I was talking to him and wondered aloud why I blew a Sentry Breath back at him. I explained that he was really overreactive, and I wanted to nip that in the bud, right here and now. If I could establish that I was to be trusted—that is, I was a bigger, better Sentry than he was—he could begin to relax. The other horses were unable to get him to trust them, and so they simply ignored his antics. For whatever reason, Brandy was not allowing the herd to guide him.

Lisa told me the bay had been gelded late due to an illness he had when he was younger, and her trainer had always thought he took on some stud-like behaviors because of this. Anything was possible, but nervous hypervigilance was more an immature response than a stallion's behavior. Seasoned stallions are supremely aware of their territory and everything in it, but they would run themselves ragged if they acted in such a way. They want to try to keep things calm instead.

For whatever reason, Brandy hadn't quite finished growing up, and he was desperately in need of a mature horse that could answer his questions and corral his anxiety. I would try to fill that role.

Starting from Behind

Lisa walked Brandy to his stall, and he nearly trampled her in the aisle. She smiled gently and stated that this was better than it used to be.

She had been practicing the Greeting ritual with Brandy and had noticed that he now came up to her more quickly and assuredly than before. He and I moved through a pleasant Greeting, and he provided some lovely Go Away Face movements himself. Lisa told me that this Button had really helped tremendously in getting him to stay calmer during halter-ing and bridling, and that his tendency to knock her over with his face was almost gone.

I noticed that as soon as we completed the Greeting and a few Go Away Face routines, along with some Sentry Breath blown toward the barn door and a couple of nice "Aw-Shucks," Brandy quickly turned around and faced his rump toward me. Lisa admitted he had been doing this for about a week, and she thought it meant he was done with the talk.

Horse the Size of a Hamster

The need to be driven is one of the most misunderstood in horses. Because of the potential for kicking, people have, understandably, made a rule of not allowing a horse turn his rump toward them, and we have become very strict about how and when to handle a horse's hind end. Brandy was in his stall and I was outside it, so I could not get kicked. When horses are hard to handle, I always use utmost caution, and I recommend people remain on the other side of a barrier for this work at first.

I could not get close enough to Brandy to touch his Hip-Drive Button, but luckily that was not necessary. As you've seen in earlier stories, pointing your finger at any Button "activates" it and asks that Button to either move or not come any closer. Pressing your palm toward a Button asks the horse to stay with you, follow you, or otherwise be connected with you.

I pointed my finger at his Hip-Drive button, and Brandy totally froze—he was not even breathing. I remained Zero, but my pointer finger had a Level 3 ("telling") intensity in it. Inside I was calm, but that pointer finger was almost on fire.

After a full minute of freezing, Brandy blew out a big releasing breath and stepped away from me in a circle in his stall. As soon as he turned back toward me, he lowered his head and flopped his ears to the side, licking and chewing.

Brandy was ready to talk. We had gone through the beginning of the Greeting ritual and the first few phases of creating space with Go Away Face and "Aw-Shucks." Now he was asking the question he most needed answered:

"Who's driving?"

AHA MOMENT

Insecure horses crave to be driven forward and protected from behind, and this is what Brandy desperately needed. But he was so large and energetic that none of the other horses in his home herd felt like doing what it would take to move him around and control him.

He was large on the outside, but inside, Brandy felt like a hamster—tiny and unprotected.

As I have worked to understand the nuances of Horse Speak, I have come to understand that the Hip-Drive Button can also be a question posed to someone. Basically, if a person feels weak, intimidated, or even just "down in the dumps," and the horse offers the Hip-Drive Button slowly and casually, he is asking the question: "Are you feeling okay?" If a horse that is normally the group's Leader is not feeling well, then the subordinates need to know that. Offering the Hip-Drive Button toward the Leader serves as a Check-In: "Are you feeling up to the job of kicking coyotes?"

Many horses will offer their rump to their trusted owner with an ulterior motive: they want their butt scratched! Oftentimes a horse loves this so much he may become quite bold about swinging his hip toward you. Even in these cases, take a moment to also use your pointer finger to say back to the horse, "Yes, I *will* scratch your butt; however, I am still in charge back here, and you need to move off if I say so." It is important.

Am I Up for This?

There have been many situations in which the work I am doing with a horse and human may reveal deeper layers of the human's personal growth or struggle. In these situations, I have witnessed horses turn around simply to ask how the person is feeling. The horse is not panicked, or needing leadership, or wanting a scratch—he is simply commenting on the fact that his beloved human seems to be feeling "off" in that moment.

I told Lisa about these different scenarios as I used Brandy's Hip-Drive Button to move him forward into a circle and then face me again three more times. After the third time, Brandy closed his eyes and needed a nap. This was good news, as it meant that he was absorbing the lesson.

I had not yet touched him.

If I had tried to do this initial work in an open paddock, riding ring, or round pen it could have easily gotten very big and out of control, because Brandy's personality was the type to quickly get overexcited. Introducing the idea in a small, quiet setting first, as we were, was ideal.

After his nap break, I told Lisa to take Brandy out of his stall. He was very quiet and helpful for the first few minutes, but he lost his composure once he was in the aisle. She said the bay always got pushy and wanted to touch everything. I told her to go ahead and let him, but she was to oversee what he could touch, and how, and when. So, Lisa went ahead and led him up to objects all along the barn aisle, chatting away about whatever it was and its function. She admitted she felt rather silly. This also went against a life's worth of equine-related training that stated, "The horse must not touch things and must be under control at all times."

However, after only about three minutes, Brandy stopped desperately tugging on the lead rope and started calmly walking with Lisa as she approached each new object. He wiggled his ears and seemed to take a real interest as she explained the items. She was so amused by this that she asked me if I thought he understood English. I don't know how many human words horses learn, but they do seem to pick up on certain ones. Really, though, it was Lisa's casual conversational tone that he was likely reacting to—it puts many, many horses at ease. I believe our body language becomes very congruent when we speak out loud, and horses find this soothing.

Soon, Brandy was yawning and rolling his shoulder blades forward so that he was off his tippy toes and looking shorter—even fatter—as he released his hind gut and started taking deep breaths.

It was time to end the session. We set up a follow-up for a month later.

Out in the Field

When I returned, Lisa met me in the driveway with a big hug. She was very pleased with how much progress Brandy had made since my last visit. He was much easier to lead and hardly ever pulled on the lead rope. He still was cautious and a bit high-strung, but gone were the regular tug-o-wars that had been part of their normal routine.

I asked Lisa if she was comfortable being out in the field with Brandy. She said she had found herself lingering with him more and more out there, so I asked her to slip through the fence into the pasture where the geldings hung out.

Immediately, Brandy made a beeline for her, stopping about 5 feet away to do an "Aw-Shucks" and Go Away Face out of respect. Lisa also looked away and blew a Sentry Breath for good measure. The bay then marched right up to her and they had a nice Greeting. She asked him to move his face and neck away, and he took initiative and stepped lightly aside with his front feet, as well. Lisa told me this was now very easy to do—it was part of their usual routine together. She felt very at ease with him on the ground these days, which was a big—and positive—change.

Brandy immediately reached down to touch Lisa's foot with his muzzle. She told me he had been doing this a lot lately, and she didn't know what it meant. I explained it was a request to step back away from his head. Once you have said hello, it is awkward for horses if you just stand around near their face. Horses buddy up at the shoulder, and this is a logical next step in conscientiously hanging out together.

Brandy blew out a big breath of release, and Lisa copied him. Then he did a sort of fast "Aw-Shucks," bobbing his head a little. She said he often did this, and she did not know what to do when he did. I explained he was requesting that they move off together. He carefully leaned away from her and took a slow, deliberate step. I told her to Copycat his movements and just "match steps" with him. She moved foot for foot when he did, and soon they were moving around the field slowly and carefully but fully engaged. Brandy challenged her to step over rocks or change direction. He stopped, dropped his nose to the ground, and turned his nose far away from her foot this time. I told her that this was a request to now move off on his own.

"Okay, Brandy…go off then," Lisa said out loud. And she swished her hand-tail to show him she was done. He swished, too, and casually walked off in the direction he had looked. She made her way back to me, beaming.

"That was so fun!" Lisa exclaimed. "I never let him lead me around before! It was so connected and…sweet."

As Lisa was walking up to me, her older mare Misty came up behind me to meet her at the fence. Before we could talk about what had happened with Brandy, Misty was commanding our attention.

Misty clearly had something to say.

The Mares Are Talking

Misty was a good-sized Appaloosa, predominantly white with some leopard spots. She reached for Lisa and the pair had a quick, three-touch Greeting, and then Misty immediately touched Lisa's feet with her nose. I told Lisa the mare wanted her feet to move, and Lisa asked how she should move them—before I could answer, Misty arranged herself delicately to place Lisa at her shoulder. Lisa smiled, and said, "Well I guess I got my answer!"

Misty then reached around to gently touch Lisa in the stomach with her nose. I told her to rearrange where her bellybutton was aiming. As Lisa turned aside, I had a flash of insight.

"Lisa, offer her a 'hug' by placing your near hand under her jaw and beckoning her face to come around your torso."

AHA MOMENT

As soon as Misty had drawn her face toward Lisa's torso, she suddenly stopped, put her ears backward, and lifted her head quite high. Lisa stood very still, and so did Misty. I asked Lisa how she was feeling at that moment, because the mare's reaction, at first willing, but then distanced, was interesting.

After some thought, Lisa admitted she felt guilty about not spending as much time with her old mare as she used to. As soon as she spoke these words, Misty reached around and "hugged" her of her own accord.

When Lisa raised her hands to embrace her mare's face, Misty pulled away again.

I asked her what she was feeling now. Lisa acknowledged she felt like she didn't deserve this affection because of her guilt. Lisa was very bold about being totally honest, and this allowed Misty to keep the conversation flowing. The mare reached around again to "hug" her. This time, Lisa told Misty out loud, "I'm sorry, I don't mean to ignore you. You really are a treasure to me."

Lisa again brought her hands up to embrace Misty's face, and now the mare hovered lightly in her arms for a moment, before carefully untangling and straightening out. Misty licked and chewed and blew out a few relaxation breaths, as did Lisa.

A Little Goes a Long Way

A few weeks later, I was back for another session. Since our last meeting, Lisa had become very aware of her energy in her core and her intention. She wondered how that would affect the other work she did with Brandy.

We brought him into the indoor arena where she rode him nearly every day. Lisa had found success "blowing away the bogeyman" in the indoor, so Brandy was much calmer than he used to be. He was still the type to look for or even invent "problems," so I wanted to help Lisa to find Zero in this environment.

I talked to Brandy about his concerns (there were plenty: the far gate, a blue barrel, the sound of cars driving by on the road), and he blew out his nose and lowered his head, flopping his ears sideways. Lisa asked about addressing specific things with Sentry Breath as she had thought you just "blow Sentry" in general, all the time. I told her that the first day, or even few days, of using Horse Speak, that is fine because you and your horse are getting used to talking about it. However, once the horse believes you will be his Sentry, he begins looking for your leadership. This allows him to transition into only asking about specific concerns. I reminded her of our first lesson in the barn where she introduced him to all the items in the aisle. This was much like that early scene: The horse that is following is watching the Leader interact with things, and then becoming brave enough to do it, too—the way he once did with his mom.

Lisa had become very good at leading Brandy with her palm down (see p. 81), anchoring her footfalls so that she took defined steps, and stopping him with one single stomp that he pulled up for every time. Now that those skills were easy, it was time to bring their core energy into the conversation (see p. 50). I asked her to move the bay out into a free-longe circle, which he was very comfortable doing. As soon as she pointed the whip at him, he moved out to the rail, following her voice commands quite nicely into walk, trot, and canter. I always like to see what people and their horses are already good at doing together—then we can simply introduce Horse Speak into the mix and take what is good to the next level of greatness.

Boring Becomes Interesting

Neither Lisa nor Brandy was overly excited about free-longeing; it was just something they did to get a little exercise. Brandy was not turning away from her or avoiding her, but he was not interested either. Her body language was simple and uncomplicated, but I could see she, too, found all this a little boring.

Lisa had brought Brandy down to a halt when I had her ask him to move up to a trot again, only this time I wanted her to *focus on her core* as she asked. I didn't want her to change anything else; just add this focus. As soon as Brandy had trotted about three steps, Lisa instinctively put her free hand on her bellybutton to think about it. This change of hand position got her horse's attention, and his ears and eyes darted toward her. I suggested she make a small "sitting motion" as though she was going to sit in a chair—the focus, however, was not on sitting, but on strengthening the awareness of her core. As soon as she attempted this, Brandy shortened his stride, but elevated it as well, using his hind end to carry and lift himself. Lisa smiled ear to ear. I told her to stand tall again, and when she did, the bay lengthened his stride and stretched his neck lower to the ground. Now I asked her to aim her core in front of his nose. He tucked backward and elevated his poll until, caught in the moment, Lisa stepped forward by accident, not realizing this would stop him. He came to an abrupt halt and turned his head to look at her with interested eyes.

She wasn't sure what had just happened, but she liked it!

I explained that when she aimed her core at his Girth Button while "sitting," this asked him to stay connected with her but change his intensity level. He accomplished this by shortening and lifting his stride. When she aimed toward his Greeting Button, he had lifted his poll to tuck his nose, replying to her request. When she stepped forward with her core energy directed to his chest, she was mimicking how one horse tells another they are about to cross paths. The subordinate horse will then "tuck back" and stop or change direction in response.

Lisa replied that because it had happened so fast, she couldn't process it in the moment. I explained that this was exactly the reason why I encouraged people to practice Horse Speak very slowly and deliberately at first. When everything is happening quickly, it is equivalent to shifting from learning a foreign language slowly, word by word, and then trying to listen to two native speakers have a conversation. Speed comes with time and practice; no one would expect a student to speak quickly within the first week of learning a new language. Horses speak with every movement they make, and more nuance becomes visible when we can stay quiet and Zero internally.

And Chew Gum

As we walked Brandy back to the barn, I asked Lisa to be consistently aware of her core as she walked him. He became agitated as she struggled to do this, so I took over, exaggerating my core energy for her to see. Imagine you are aiming a hose at a garden: The water is shooting out of your core and hitting whatever you look at. "Turning down" the core energy is like shutting the hose off.

Brandy responded well and began focusing on whatever I was focusing on instead of the whole wide world, like he usually did. Lisa took him back and tried to copy me, but again, he became frustrated with her.

I felt he was not confident enough in himself for her to learn something new with him at the same time. So we took out Misty, who had shown herself to be not only able to handle Lisa's learning curve, but interested in it, as well.

I began, taking Misty's lead rope and "opening" my core energy for her to follow. In a matter of moments, she had lowered her head and was licking and chewing, with her ears sideways and her focus completely on whatever I was looking at. She not only enjoyed this clarity of focus but approved! I walked across the grass, then I stopped, aiming my core on a patch of nice green growth. Misty hesitated, wanting a Check-In with my knuckles first, then gladly ate the tender shoots. I turned the "hose" off and stood there casually. When a car drove past, I aimed my core at it, and protectively placed my palm toward the mare much the way a parent places a child in behind her before crossing the street. Misty responded by immediately tucking in behind me and raising her head for a moment to look at the car. We both breathed out and relaxed, agreeing that it was just a car, after all. I asked her to lift her head and walk off with me, and she elegantly fulfilled this request with her nose blowing and eyes blinking. We walked farther with her slightly behind me, her head low, both of us taking deep, sauntering steps. We stopped together next to Lisa as though we were in a waltz and each synchronized movement was choreographed.

"First of all," Lisa said, "I have *never* seen her willingly leave a clump of grass. Second, she is notorious for walking very fast, like she is on a mission. You usually get the feeling that she is in charge, and you better keep up."

Your Turn

I handed Lisa the lead rope and told her to try and copy the whole thing. She struggled to keep control of her core energy while also leading her horse. Luckily, our bodies are hard-wired to create a feeling based on whatever posture we are in. I told her to find "O" posture first, then to extend her leading hand forward as though she had a hose nozzle in it when she began leading. I explained she should keep her knees more bent in her walk because bent knees require the abdomen to engage differently, and thus keep some of your attention there by default. We tend to stand straight up when leading horses with no awareness of our core at all, instead focusing on our arms and hands as we use the lead rope. My first solution to this is to bring awareness to the feet by "Matching Steps" (see p. 136). This begins to inform the connection between horse and human by engaging the person's lower half. As we learned earlier (see p. 81), turning the palms down on the lead then sends an anchoring and grounding sensation to our own brains, as well as to the horse. The last (and typically most difficult) step is actually engaging the core. When all the other body parts are more present, engaging the core is the last and deepest part of the conversation.

It took Lisa a few minutes to orchestrate this effect, but as soon as she found it, the result was unmistakable. Misty instantly dropped her head, relaxed her ears, and dropped back a step to adopt the following position behind Lisa. Lisa was so empowered by this that she strutted right over to the grass, selecting a nice patch for Misty the way I had. The mare looked for a Check-In first, then happily ate the grass. Lisa felt like she was off the hook and began to eagerly outline what she was experiencing. Misty put an end to this, however—suddenly, Lisa was being dragged to another grassy spot, as Misty slipped the rope over her shoulder in the position that clever horses figure out, which allows them to have real leverage against the human.

Lisa fell back into what was most familiar, tugging back at her, calling, "Hey there!" I told her to instead move toward Misty's face in her "O" posture, taking the tension out of the rope and asking the horse to reconnect. Misty stopped pulling and lifted her head to touch her nose to Lisa's hands, flipping her tail in an exaggerated manner.

I took Misty and demonstrated how my posture held more of an "X" pose the whole time with my core energy focused on what we were doing, even if I turned to talk to Lisa. This made Misty feel included and held in place instead of "turned loose" with the lack of attention.

Lisa admitted she hadn't realized that being distracted when in her horse's presence made the horse feel "turned loose."

"That makes perfect sense," she agreed. "If I am completely focused on her, then take that away, my body language is saying she is free to do as she pleases. I wonder how often I am leading a horse, but I am distracted? I can see where that would be really frustrating for a horse to have constant mixed messages."

It was time to go get Brandy again to see if her new awareness could change that relationship.

The Proof Is in the Brandy

As she led Brandy out of the barn, Lisa paid attention to every single step. She also focused her core energy, and allowed time to consider any objects that he found interesting or challenging (like the threshold of the barn door, for instance). Brandy moved with concentration and care, and a much lower head than usual. When she stopped, he stopped quickly alongside her and held perfectly still. She was amazed that he could carry such a degree of concentration, seeing as he had always been a flighty, distractible horse.

Lisa also found the intense level of focus a bit tiring! I laughed and said that was why the other horses didn't want to give Brandy what he really needed. Her herd of relaxed retirees did not have the energy to school the worried youngster, but if Lisa did, he would mature very rapidly.

I suggested she use the next few weeks to apply this hyper-focus to *every-thing* they did on the ground. Interestingly, because they did dressage, Brandy seemed to have this need mostly filled while under saddle: There was so much focus and concentration from Lisa when she rode him that he was feeling nurtured there. But Brandy needed to feel this kind of care throughout the rest of his life.

The Herd at Zero

When I saw Lisa at an event a few weeks later, she reported that it was like Brandy's entire work ethic had an overhaul. Not only was he more attentive under saddle, but all the groundwork they did—even just tacking him up—had become an exercise in awareness that surprised and delighted her. One of the benefits had also been that the bay was much less pushy with the other horses. And, the rest of the herd was also including Lisa in their world more so than before. It was as if everyone on the property had taken a deep breath and were now so much more comfortable with each other.

The whole herd was going to Zero. The herd as an entity wants to live in this state, so when one horse or human goes there, they will all find their way.

Lisa also reported that she had taken Misty out for a few trail rides as they had rekindled their relationship. The Appy was still telling Lisa when she was tense or "off" in any way, but now Lisa looked forward to these comments, because she was truly dedicated to being as clear as she could with her herd. She said that sometimes something would happen between herself and Brandy that was a little confusing, and now she knew to go right over to Misty and tell her about it. Somehow, Misty always seemed to help her feel her Zero again, and sometimes the mare would do something that seemed to serve to advise Lisa about what to do.

Lisa acknowledged that a part of her still had a hard time believing this was really happening, but her daily interactions were becoming so full of valuable conversations that it was as though her fluency in Horse Speak was outdistancing her disbelief. Her horses were communicating with her, and although it was not perfect, it was a lot of fun!

LICK AND CHEW

Horses who act out frequently desire to have their hind-end protected. In fact, I can almost guarantee that an insecure horse will show me his Hip-Drive Button at some point in this predictable, low-impact manner. All too often, high-energy horses that we wish to cultivate advanced levels of riding with also have more complex needs. By assuring Brandy I would "kick the coyotes," I was able to get a grip on his insecurities. Spending quality time reassuring a horse from the hind end can do quite a lot for increasing his confidence. Always be mindful, however, of a horse's defensive end. It is for this reason that I began work with Brandy from *outside* his stall, with him inside, and a door between us.

Many of us feel guilty for not having enough time to spend with our horses. We are so busy in our daily lives, this is not uncommon. However, it was only when Lisa could release that guilt that she could find the extra "oomph" she needed to add power to her core energy and truly lead her horses.

Chapter 12

Healer Horses Getting Healed

I was offered an opportunity to collaborate with a local psychotherapist who saw individual clients and occasionally did EMDR (eye movement desensitization and reprocessing) on horseback. Sara had been not only providing horse-assisted psychotherapy for many years, but also taught and certified equine specialists—those who handle the horses and look out for their best interest in any therapeutic program that works with horses.

Sara had a mare with a traumatic history: Something happened to her while being trailered to a new farm when she was very young, and when she arrived, she was blind. Sara didn't know exactly what happened—just that this strange trauma had occurred. The mare had then panicked in the new environment (before anyone realized what had happened), broke loose, and ended up tangled in some old wire in the woods. Although she was tended to with care after the incident, she didn't fare well and was eventually deemed a lost cause and sent out to pasture. Eventually she found her way to Sara, who was determined to at least give Bonnie, as she called her, the best life possible.

Bonnie was a sweet mare in a lot of ways, but at 16 hands, she was tough to deal with if she got panicky. Over the years, her eyesight had seemed to level out and she had even regained some, although she still needed a lot of coaxing in and out of doors.

Recently, Bonnie had "volunteered" to work with a few of Sara's clients. Sara deemed it "volunteering" because when she approached her herd, usually one of the horses would come over and to be with her and the client. Since this work simply involved someone grooming Bonnie or standing near her while she grazed, Sara saw this as doable and an improvement in the horse's comfort level.

Let Me Help You

I first met Bonnie while assisting Sara during a session with one of her clients. Bonnie seemed to catch on to the fact that my role was narrating what I could interpret from her body language to the client. Sara later stated that normally, Bonnie did very little during the sessions, and she and the client simply used the proximity of the horse to add a level of comfort and awareness to the therapeutic process. Sara also said the mare sought very little contact in general. However, with my narration, Bonnie became much more active, seeking contact, and even changing directions, which placed the client's hands on different zones as the horse tried to communicate more clearly. To be clear: Bonnie was not seeking a scratch or stroke. What she was doing was leaning into the client's touch, holding very steady, providing "positive" physical feedback. I did my best to speak for her, and each time the client had a moment of insight based on what was being said, the mare blew out a deep breath, lowered her head, or changed positions.

After about 60 minutes had passed, Bonnie politely left us and walked away, causing Sara to look at her watch and agree that it had been an hour, the session was over.

We all chuckled.

From Nightmare to Fresh Start

The next week, Sara asked if I would just work with Bonnie. I agreed as I was fascinated by her backstory and the previous week's actions, so we brought Bonnie into her stall to allow her to feel comfortable and to enable us to focus on her alone without the whole herd around.

Sara told me that one of the difficult aspects of living with Bonnie was that her emotional range was all over the place. She would seem to be fine or even "happy," then suddenly pin her ears and try to get away for "no reason." In addition, she seemed to crave to be near Sara—lingering around whenever Sara was doing chores, rather than being out with the herd—but as soon as Sara needed to lead Bonnie anywhere, a great deal of stressful energy was produced. Sara called it "scared and angry at the same time." Bonnie never hurt anyone—she would freeze rather than run someone over—but that freeze felt very, very intense. Half of Sara wanted to get a handle on the behavior because it felt chaotic, but the other half just felt like she was missing something vital about how to help the sweet mare.

With all the best intentions from both the horse and her human, the way back was still just a little elusive.

Since Sara and I had both gone over the full Greeting ritual with Bonnie when I first came to the farm, I wasn't sure what she would want to do. As soon as I approached the stall, Bonnie did a Check-In then a Go Away Face, then brought her muzzle back for number two. This told me that she wanted the formality of the full ritual. We completed the third Greeting, and I stepped away. She also stepped away in a respectful Copycat, then she made one full turn in her stall and came back to the front with her face away from me and the door. I had come to recognize that when a horse does this quiet turn around, he is showing me all his buttons and offering to really communicate. The signal Bonnie used to show me it was all right to enter the stall was holding her head to the side, away from the door. A horse that holds his head right at the door is asking to leave. When a horse turns around and stands steadily with his rump to you—looking backward a little to see you, maybe—he is suggesting you communicate with his Hip-Drive Button. However, if when he turns his rump toward you he hides his head in a corner or against a wall, cocks a foot, or swishes a tail—he is done.

Sara and I entered the stall, and Bonnie stood very still. Sara was interested in learning about the Buttons and what each seemed to mean, so I held my palm at each Button to see how Bonnie felt about connecting with me at each one (see p. 42 for a refresher of where the Buttons are located). As soon as I held my palm to the Go Away Face button (which, remember, essentially says, "Don't go away, stay with me here,") Bonnie seemed to stiffen up. She did not do anything negative, but by getting tense, I could see she had a problem with the request. We were just gathering information, so this didn't worry me. Moving down to the Mid-Neck Button, Bonnie tensed up again, this time lifting her head a little higher. I moved down to her Shoulder Button and she remained the same, but not worse. Lingering at her Girth Button, I offered a deep breath. Suddenly, she shuddered and lowered her head, licking and chewing.

How interesting!

Moving my palms down to the Jump-Up Button, I filled my whole ribcage with air, and so did Bonnie. We remained in this position for a few minutes, then I finished by holding my palm first to the Hip-Drive Button and lastly the

Yield-Over Button in the hollow of the stifle. For the two buttons on her hind end, she was very calm and steady.

Sara then stepped in to do the same thing as I had done, to see if Bonnie reacted any differently with her own person. Bonnie gave roughly the same response, all the way through. Sara and I stepped outside to think about this. The horse blew out her nose, shook her neck, and stood in the back corner of her stall with a foot cocked.

Think-Tank

Sara's specialty was working with people with traumatic backgrounds. Since we both knew that Bonnie *had* a traumatic background, we started correlating her responses to what Sara called "stored memories." Since Bonnie could not actually tell us about her memories or if she was remembering the past or conditioned to feel reactive in those areas now—or both—we needed to come up with a way to see if we could help her feel more comfortable around her front end.

Blindness caused by head trauma, some sort of mysterious trailering incident, breaking through fencing in a brand-new environment, and then getting tangled up in wire in the woods all qualified this horse for some sort of post-traumatic stress disorder (PTSD). Having worked with horses suffering from similar issues for many years at rescues, it was wonderful to have a skilled human therapist who could "think-tank" with me now about Bonnie and what we were experiencing. I have had enough practice to "trust my gut" about how to go forward in these situations but usually have little to no background for the horse. Sara could help because, although she specialized in humans, not horses, all mammals have similar freeze mechanisms and when exposed to prolonged stress and animals exhibit signs of PTSD, just like humans; we know this because scientists have induced stress in laboratory animals to study the effects on the brain. Zoos now provide "enrichment" protocols because zookeepers became aware that the pacing, frantic energy, or depressed, aberrant behaviors they witnessed in zoo animals were stress-induced.

So, where to begin? We went back into the stall, and this time I activated the Buttons, either asking them to move over or asking them to lean toward me. Bonnie was okay moving over but did not want to draw near me in the front end. Her girth, belly, and hind end were fine.

Sara stated that when working with a human client, she would help her find a "safe space," in order to have a baseline to come back to if the therapy got too intense. What would Bonnie's safe space be? Although Bonnie didn't seek touch with her front end, she was very comfortable with her hind end being touched—even now seeking some scratching there—we decided that would be one area to which we could retreat to maintain contact, but give her some ease.

It occurred to me that the Tai Chi move "roll the ball" might serve as a way to connect on a deeper level with Bonnie. This is a warm-up in which you stand with your feet apart, "holding the ball" as we discussed on page 75 over one knee. You make a large, slow, round motion as though you are rolling the ball from in front of your chin all the way out and down toward your bellybutton. This cultivates deep relaxation and is supposed to be restorative. Sara and I did it in front of Bonnie for a minute, and then took turns massaging her hind end with the same rolling, downward focus that was rhythmic and soothing. The mare began to rock with the rhythm, and then closed her eyes and drooped her lips.

Stepping out of the stall, we allowed Bonnie to absorb what had just happened. We wanted to see if we had helped create a "safe spot" for her.

Offering Healing

Sara and I went back into the stall and again offered to touch our palms to Bonnie, who now stood very still and seemed more grounded. Her feet were all lined up square, in balance, her breathing was deep and relaxed, and her face was softer. She tolerated our palms pressing the Buttons much better, and Sara simply spoke quietly about what she knew Bonnie had been through and that whatever Bonnie needed to be or to feel about that was fine with her. She then stopped talking and practiced her Zero. Sara was a whiz at Zero, since she needed to be able to regularly "get there" for her work as a therapist. I reminded Sara that since she already had such a deep wealth of experience and expertise in the world of trauma, she could bring those skills to mind whenever dealing with Bonnie. She didn't need to only rely on "horse-handling" techniques, especially those that were not making as much progress.

This time, when Sara reached for Bonnie's Girth Button, the mare shifted herself so that she could reach around and touch her muzzle to Sara's arm very gently. I suggested Sara back up to her shoulder and hold her hands out into a welcoming "O" for Bonnie to reach into. This was the horse "hug" position. Horses also like to stand shoulder to shoulder and hang their necks across each other from time to time.

There was a lovely, warm feeling in the air as the two of them became lost in a soft embrace. For this mare to offer a "hug" was no small thing. Sara had all the feel and timing she needed to hold the embrace lightly but not ask for more, and she let it go as soon as the horse was done. When it was over, Bonnie carefully stepped forward until Sara was at her hip, and then she seemed to droop her hind end down to ask for contact. Sara did "roll the ball" to her rump again, and for the first few moments, Bonnie nervously chewed on the wood in her stall. Sara wondered aloud what that was about—it was my feeling that the closeness in that "hug" encounter was almost too much for Bonnie, and she was relieving stress and had sent her person to her safe spot, to boot.

AHA MOMENT

Whether Bonnie recognized contact with her rump as a safe spot or simply had enjoyed the experience and wanted it again wasn't clear. The important point here was she could have just as easily moved away, swished her tail, and asked to be done. I had been in situations like this dozens of times before and witnessed horses make similar choices—that is, opting for connection and help rather than disconnection and isolation.

A Good Cry

Sara and I again stepped out into the aisle. Now that she could take her "therapy hat" off, tears of joy slipped out. Sara felt that Bonnie had "chosen" her somehow in that moment. Prior to this, they had basically enjoyed each other's company, but the horse was so standoffish and temperamental that Sara could not feel a real deep connection to the mare.

Sara's work was very much about helping people come into the present and become comfortable in their own bodies again. In essence, she was restoring Zero to her clients. We discussed how, in a human process, we use talking to help a person face and release past issues, but when you are trying to help a horse you cannot use words.

Bonnie had become more embodied as we worked with her, and she had been willing to go into what troubled her as we progressed, calmly and predictably. That is why Sara chose to end our session at that point. I agreed that we should end there and not try to do more. I thought the "horse hug" had been a significant invitation. It was time to let it be.

Sara wanted to give Bonnie a little exercise going forward, but leading, longeing, liberty—they all tended to make her more tense rather than the other way around. It was all related to how hard it was for the mare to deal with anything about her front end (remember her initial reaction to our palms on her Buttons). But, then again, you could safely pick up all four feet, and she was extremely careful, even in panicky moments, to never run anyone over or hurt anyone.

I told Sara that if she was going to try to reach Bonnie while loose in a pen, she would need to repeat all the same things we had done in the stall. If Bonnie was so tense in the pen that Sara didn't feel safe inside with her, then she should still try to go through the steps from outside the pen. If it was possible, I recommended again establishing a safe spot inside the pen before turning her loose. Then, if she got to a place where she felt it was time to ask the mare to walk out a little bit, she should ask for three changes of direction and call it a day. Horses use (in general) three changes of direction to curb big ideas or big feelings, or change their mind, or try to change another horse's mind. (This is why, like I've mentioned before, I might make three changes of direction while pacing outside a pen or stall before I approach a timid or difficult horse.)

Chosen by Bonnie

Not long after, I heard from Sara that she had tried a light exercise session in the pen with Bonnie. The whole way out to the pen was tense, and even revisiting the mare's safe spot with a rub on her rump did little to relax her. But Bonnie allowed it. When Sara turned her loose in the pen, Bonnie took off in full flight, so Sara decided to stay outside the pen.

To help cue the three changes of direction, Sara had a flag tied to a stick. As Bonnie came careening past her once, Sara lifted the flag up and wiggled it in front of the motion. Now, Sara and her flag were on the outside, and Bonnie could have easily just ignored them both and sailed past, but she reacted like she hit a brick wall, digging her heels into the ground for an all-out rollback. The second pass and turn was a little easier, and after the third change of direction, Sara sat down in the grass and laid down the flag to let Bonnie know that was it, they were done. Bonnie trotted around a bit, blowing Sentry Breath, which Sara answered with her own. Then, Bonnie did an interesting thing. She slowed to a walk, then finally a halt, and turned her rump toward Sara, drooping it down in the "please come scratch me" position. Sara wasted no time, and went right in to greet her hind end and rub her gently in her safe spot.

By the time Sara put the halter and lead rope on to take her back to the barn, Bonnie had flopped her ears to the side and was closing her eyes and drooping her lips. She was relaxed and anchoring each step. Sara "Matched Steps" with her and stopped her feet every 10 feet or so to see what Bonnie did. Bonnie stopped along with her, every time, without once pulling for grass or acting in the least bit ruffled. It was like a light bulb had gone off for them both.

Sometimes, all it takes is three changes of direction for something different to show up. It is simple enough thing to try.

Two Hearts as One

A few weeks later, I was back at Sara's house, practicing the Tai Chi "roll the ball" move again. The horses were all out in the field, and we stood in the paddock area near the barn. The paddock had an open gate, so the horses could come check us out if they wanted to.

As we "rolled the ball," I suggested that Sara think of offering her heart out when her hands went out, and then scooping up heart energy when she brought her hands back in. Sara grinned and said, funny I mention it, because this was the lesson she felt she was getting from Bonnie more and more: that of giving and receiving heart energy.

She had no sooner said it than Bonnie whinnied loudly from way up in the back field. Thundering hooves made a beeline for us, and soon Bonnie rounded the corner, stopped to stare at us for a minute, then sauntered down to the paddock to stand nearby, cocking a hip and lowering her head. Sara wanted to move to her with the open-heart feeling she had developed in her rhythmic motion of "roll the ball." Bonnie allowed herself to be touched all over—she did not want too much around her head and neck, but did not completely tense up there, either.

Both of us got a bit misty-eyed because the sensitivity and kindness emanating from Bonnie was so clear.

In a few short weeks, Bonnie was beginning to find a deep relaxation in everything she did. Her interest in being involved with Sara's clients was quite amazing—she was the horse that "volunteered" most often. Best of all, Sara gained so much trust in her, she started doing some light riding. Any time Bonnie got nervous, Sara would reach behind her and scratch the mare's rump. Bonnie would pause and take a big breath—and keep trying.

LICK AND CHEW

By using the Horse Speak Buttons as a diagnostic tool, we came to a better understanding of Bonnie's "stuck" places. By bringing concentrated awareness to these areas, new insights that eventually led to breakthroughs were possible.

I am always amazed at the ability and desire of horses to offer such compassion to human beings. With enough calm presence, awareness, and willingness, any person can bring healing to a horse in need with more ease than you might think.

What a gift that horses seek to offer this right back to us.

Chapter 13

Brand New Old Friends

In southern Vermont where I live, there is a horsewoman who is well known for her thoughtful horsemanship. Her career has led her down many of the same interesting paths I have been on, so when we met face to face, there was such harmony between us that we instantly knew we wanted to spend more time together.

After only a few sessions practicing Horse Speak, Heidi said, "This is like the ground floor underneath all the other stuff. If you can speak the language, then whatever you want to do is automatically enhanced."

Heidi and I began collaborating and working together to help other professionals learn the basics. She was interested in applying Horse Speak to riding principles, and I was excited to have such a talented rider and riding instructor to work with. Of course, Horse Speak applies whether you are standing on the ground or sitting on the horse's back, but frequently, once the relationship on the ground becomes better, the riding improves naturally. People find themselves "blowing away the bogeyman," or doing a Shuddering Breath, or using other aspects of Horse Speak without a second thought.

Heidi's own horse, a Cheval Canadien named Riley, was a nice guy. Having grown up with Heidi, he was friendly and open and eager to learn. However, Riley had a few "Riley-isms" that were quirky and had caused his owner to pause and scratch her head on many occasions. She found out that when he was two days old, he had yet to lie down! Even the vet was concerned; he proclaimed the little guy could die from exhaustion and so helped him find his way to the ground to rest. As a foal, Riley had also once been so afraid of crossing a narrow ditch to follow his mom he had begun to panic. His owners at the time literally had to carry him across so that he could join her.

Riley got "stuck" when he couldn't figure something out, and now that he was a huge horse, you couldn't just physically move him to get him sorted out.

The level of intensity it would take to get him going when he was stuck was not the way Heidi chose to work her horses; she wanted to find another answer.

Otherwise, Riley was totally responsive.

What a conundrum!

After using Horse Speak for a few months, Heidi and Riley had sorted out certain things on the ground. She wanted to see what Horse Speak could do for their riding.

Pivot Points

I watched Heidi and Riley together through all the steps of tacking up, pre-mounting, and mounting. We paused at any little spot where there seemed to be confusion for Riley and worked together to help him understand better. By the time Heidi was ready to get on, we almost needed a break!

I told her to just go ahead and go through her normal warm-up and riding session. I always like to see what is already working for a horse-and-rider pair. And I honestly thought just about everything *was* working between Heidi and Riley. They knew each other so well.

But there was one little thing that kept showing up which both Heidi and her dressage coaches had noticed and worked on: Riley was not that relaxed in his ribs. He was otherwise generally "relaxed and forward," but he sometimes seemed to not be using himself to the fullest. My eye could see that the Girth Button and Jump-Up button were not really engaged (see p. 42 for an illustration of the 13 Buttons). When this is the case, a horse will often look "tucked up," inhibited, or will shorten his stride. His bends and circles will be just a little "off," because if a horse cannot fully use his own internal natural pivot point (the center around which he rotates), he has to compensate by adapting in other ways. Amazingly, a horse can actually pivot from *any* of the Buttons by means of translating a turn or bend through a change of awareness and balance in that zone of his body. You can see this in a natural setting as a horse rears, bucks, rolls back, or runs over rugged terrain. Through the in-depth work I had done previously with my horse Dakota, I had come to have a tremendous understanding of how horses often orient themselves toward a single Button and balance all their movement from that point. My eye is always watching for which Button a horse is comfortable or uncomfortable with.

Certain exercises seemed to help Riley for a while, but he would then fall back into his old pattern. He had regular chiropractic and acupuncture, and his saddle was specially fit to him. Heidi often rode him bitless, but the issue cropped up whether or not he had a bit in his mouth. Overall Riley was a nice mover, and he was usually compliant and willing. Heidi used a lot of deep breathing and was a soft, lovely rider. So what was missing?

At first I was not at all sure what I could add to the equation, but I knew it wouldn't hurt to apply the body language that Rocky had taught me to the situation to see if Riley might be able to tell us something. To begin using body language instead of traditional riding cues, I suggested Heidi change the way she held the reins so her palms were down on the reins, just like I use when leading a horse (see p. 81). In about three strides, Riley stretched out his neck and gained "roominess" in his front end—it looked like his lower neck and shoulders had deeply released and begun to extend with his forehand in a rhythmic sort of swagger. He started blowing out deep breaths. Heidi leaned over toward his neck and took a deep inhaling sniff of his mane. She had sniffed his neck on the ground before riding, and he seemed to swoon from it there. Just as before, Riley's face became what could be described as "gleeful": He flopped his ears sideways and blew his nose in response to her gesture.

The forward, roomy swagger was different from his normal walk. Heidi often took him out on a trail ride and gave him his head. He knew how to extend and reach down in the bridle to release his neck while being ridden. But that was not what this was…this was not his training, but his authentic, corresponding, physical response to Heidi's body language. Heidi and Riley were "talking" about his front end and sorting out where his "happy place" was. She could instantly tell the difference in how he moved. At the very least, Riley was communicating back to Heidi immediately and displaying many signs of deep relaxation and connection to his rider that were different from those of their usual working relationship.

Heidi wanted to keep going, so I suggested we ask Riley to use his Mid-Neck Button as his pivot point. In translating Rocky's lessons to many other horse and rider combinations through the years, it had become apparent that horses enjoy finding a new level of relaxation in their necks at the Mid-Neck Button—relaxation that is not forced or controlled, but rather invited. When a horse can begin a ride by using his neck as the ballast it *normally* serves him when he is on his own, it is easier to then go through the other Buttons all in a row and come to a new understanding and awareness for both horse and rider. Each Button can create a bend, yield, softening, or pivot. It requires thoughtful, conscientious engagement of each one, preferably in sequence, to be clear and direct. Since Riley seemed to be somewhat stuck in the area of the Girth and Jump-Up Buttons, starting with the Mid-Neck would allow him to have some success before we got into what might be troubling him.

Turning the hands so the palms are down on the reins while drawing one hand away from the horse's neck at about the level of the Mid-Neck Button helps the horse use his neck as a ballast under a rider. Riley's answer to this invitation was to reach comfortably into the serpentine Heidi was outlining for him. He opened his shoulders naturally and stretched out from his chest so that his entire forehand appeared to become more confident as he used himself better in the exercise. Heidi sat passively while Riley sorted out a different orientation of his own front end. Gradually, he shifted his center of balance to his girth line, directly under Heidi, and she began to have the sensation of his body lifting up and into her all by itself. I suggested that she take some deep breaths, and Riley responded by opening up his floating ribs, which I could see move from where I stood and Heidi could feel as a lovely sensation beneath her. It was like his whole body was coming together somehow. As she had been riding the serpentines and allowing Riley to use his Mid-Neck Button as his pivot point, she had also been feeling her own ribcage open up, naturally, and her neck and shoulders were corresponding in feel and movement with Riley's. As Heidi blended with her horse's body, she admitted feeling very relaxed and open, in a new and different way.

Getting the "Scoop"

I had Heidi ride figure eights and serpentines, intermingled with periodic rests, along the straight lines of the arena. Riley's pace picked up a little, and he responded well to the sense of openness the exercises encouraged. After feeling "freed" in his front end, his breathing was taking on a softer, more relaxed rhythm. I next wanted to use the "scoop" maneuver (see p. 80) to ask Riley to think about engaging his pelvis.

I had her create the "scoop" with one hand at a time, just like I used when on the ground. In this motion when riding, you "scoop" the rein in and toward your bellybutton, but you use your entire arm, all the way to your wing bone (shoulder blade). The rotation in the arm bones while riding creates an anchoring movement through your torso to your opposite hip. The whole effect is that your skeleton uses its own natural, internal pivot point to line up opposite sides, resulting in a deep inner balance. At first it didn't really matter which hand Heidi used, because we were not trying to make Riley do anything; we were exploring the effect Heidi's skeleton had on her horse's skeleton. We were also exploring Heidi's own inner relationship to oppositional forces that balanced her skeleton, from the big toe on one side of her body across to her opposite thumb. By turning her thumb outward completely, she was sure to engage the rotation of the humerus, which was essential in rotating the scapula on the same side. This rotation, in turn, affected the many subtle muscles and tendons that fed into the center of her body and across to the opposite hip, while "lightening" the hip of the same side. That opposite leg, then, was automatically engaged to create absolute balance. The horse's response would be to align himself in accordance with her position.

This may sound complicated, but it is only because I am trying to describe what is normally an unconscious balancing act that your brain performs *for* you. When you are thrown off balance while walking down the street, your body unconsciously moves to try to save you from falling. This is why your arms and legs swing in opposite directions as you walk: left hand, right foot, and vice versa—so one side of the body can "be there" to save the other if necessary. By engaging this set of body mechanics while riding, your body centers and anchors; you are moving with deeper awareness of what body mechanics does if left to itself. Typically, a new rider's subconscious reaction to losing balance on horseback is to grip and cling in the way we see a baby primate clinging to its mother. (Unfortunately, we do not have prehensile tails or gripping toes, so this doesn't work out so well for us.) I found that by teaching brand new riding students how to use their body mechanics *from day one*, their instincts shifted quickly, and their innate body wisdom could kick in so they could steady themselves without clinging.

Because I worked with students with learning disabilities for so long, I had to work around the usual teaching technique of simply calling out things to do while riding, like: "Get your heels down!" "Engage the outside rein." "Use your inside leg aid." "Sit down in your seat." Directions like these were a learning disability student's nightmare. My entire way of teaching and coaching riding became simple, direct, and aimed at setting the students' own bodies up to "trick nature" into getting that unconscious balancing act working for them. If their "lizard brain" (the section of brain that corresponds directly with the limbic system and cannot be reasoned with—it can only be conditioned) was not being triggered into survival mode because the basics of their most primal body mechanics were set up for modeling good balance on horseback, then the other parts of their brain were more available for learning. And when this was the case, their body language was telling the horse simply, "I'm fine and balanced. How are you?"

Heidi was very self-aware and had already practiced the "scoop" motion on the ground so within two strides Riley engaged his inside hind leg in response to Heidi "scooping" her inside hand. She noted she could feel how the scooping motion went all the way through her. Riley slightly arched his spine, and the power of his haunches started to roll up from behind her.

Heidi was dedicated to the art of riding and had worked with the concept of collection—finding ways to help the horse draw his body together like a giant spring, carrying more weight on the hind legs than the front legs—for many years. I say the "concept" of collection, because there are quite a few schools of thought about how to accomplish collection out there: some are terrific and others hurt the horse. Riley normally took a bit of warm up before he could start to really lift his back, bring his hind legs under his body, and flex at the poll. She was delighted to feel that this was now happening in a few strides and that Riley seemed to be initiating it, because other than "scooping" her hand and allowing her body to accept the balance this created, she was still pretty much riding passively. She was not trying to get Riley to do anything; what he was offering felt like it was his idea.

As Heidi rode the "scoop" through more figure eights and serpentines, Riley became much more forward. Every so often, she would drop the reins and let him just walk out. Finally, I asked her to go out on the rail and "scoop" both reins at the same time, using the awareness of her core and allowing her leg aids to flow along naturally with what her body wanted to do.

In a few more steps, Riley sat back over his haunches and lifted his chest. When a horse collects, it is not only his core strength that needs to engage, but the base of his neck must lift higher, with his shoulders rising upward. This creates the appearance that the horse is built "uphill." The last piece of collection is the poll arching. An arched poll can be achieved without the base of the neck lifting, but that collapses the horse's frame and leads to problems.

Heidi rode the "wave" that was beneath her for a few minutes, then slowed Riley to a walk and gave him the reins. Any new exercise with a horse needs to be presented in small doses. I can relate this to yoga class: The first time I try a new asana, I lose my composure quickly as the muscles involved tax out. However, if I correctly practice the asana, my body can develop quickly, and soon I can hold that pose longer and longer with ease.

Now What?

Heidi enjoyed working with Riley in this way and adapted the hand and arm positions to very refined motions in no time. (When I first teach these body mechanics, there needs to be room for big, gross motor skills as your whole body and mind are reconnecting the wiring toward the body's innate way of going.) She felt like the exercises had helped and Riley was gaining ground in his balance and freedom of movement. Heidi competed in Western Dressage, and she'd found the common theme in judges' comments was that Riley needed to be more forward and bend more through the rib cage. Two other dressage trainers had been helping the pair, and it still seemed like Riley could find the desired forwardness and bend sometimes, but sometimes not. It was a bit of a barn joke, "How many trainers does it take to get Riley going?"

Heidi wondered if it was just one of those "Riley-isms."

Integrating the Herd

Heidi had a neighbor who had boarded her horse with her a few years back. The little black Morgan (named "Timor") was one of those "into everything" horses. He was like the little brother tagging along, asking endless questions. Mike, the draft-horse-cross Mentor of Heidi's herd, had endlessly driven Timor around, rearing and chasing, but never harming him. Normally Mike was very quiet, but he seemed intent on putting Timor in his place.

Heidi and Timor's owner got him going under saddle and he really enjoyed it. He was fun to teach, but the truth was, he didn't always seem to know his place with people, either. There was not a mean bone in his body, but he would maybe have been better off as a lap dog.

AHA MOMENT

Having had some nice experiences, we both decided that I should get on Riley. This allowed Heidi to see him in action, which was helpful to gaining a full picture. Riley was a kind, easy-going horse, and I decided to ride him bareback so I could feel his muscle and skeleton move beneath me. I took him through the exercises Heidi had just done, and he recreated the same openness and flexion that he'd had while Heidi was on him. She knew it had felt good, but it helped her to see it, as well. She often had someone video their rides at shows so she could review them afterward, so Heidi knew what Riley usually looked like. The body language conversations we were having with him (including a fair amount of sniffing toward his neck, which seemed to really please him) were gaining Riley's interest. He was thoughtfully engaged with us and ready to interpret our movements.

In the interest of making sure I was still blending my body with his, I took a break from doing anything and just allowed myself to be with him in whatever way he wished to move. As he walked it out, he let go of all the "work" and sauntered around in his own way *and that was when I felt it*. We knew that Riley got "stuck" when he didn't know or understand some-thing, and it seemed to me that sometime, long ago when he was first learn-ing to be ridden, he stiffened the muscles around the few vertebrae directly beneath the rider. This had likely become a habit when he was first worked under saddle. When I allowed Riley to carry me in the way he wanted, he reverted to this stiffness. I could tell it was an ingrained habit, because there was no sense of emotional tension in him. It was his "normal."

This was *so* slight a feeling that Heidi was just used to it. Once I pointed it out, however, she got on and felt it for herself. Now it stood out like a sore thumb! So, what could we do about it? This was at least a clue about why Riley could sometimes move out nicely and other times lag. If his own habit was to brace there, he didn't even know he was doing it.

I got back on Riley and allowed my own spine to turn in total motion like an undulating snake, to see if he could copy me. This just made him wiggle (not what we were looking for!). So next I simply deepened my "O" posture while on his back.

That did it. He unlocked those back muscles and lifted his back slightly. I was not asking for anything else through rein or leg aids, just his back.

However, riding around in an "O" also caused him to lift his belly and use his core to carry me forward. Since we had been doing the body language balance work, it all came together in a big Riley "Aha!" moment: He snorted, shook his head, and flopped his ears to the side. Striding forward without hesitation, he found his way.

Heidi hopped on to recreate Riley's new "happy place," forming an exaggerated "O," and her horse licked and chewed and blew out his nose. He agreed that this felt better! Heidi practiced refining the "O" posture until it was just a certain level of "feel" she attained in her ribcage and belly. The pair looked beautiful. Now, just making the "O" posture helped recreate all the body language balance work we had just taken the time to practice. Riley was invested in Heidi's requests because he was taking "ownership" over the final product, so to speak. It was not just Heidi telling Riley how to move, but Riley feeling better within himself, having sorted out something that was confusing.

Heidi and Riley competed at a Western Dressage show that weekend, and they received the highest points they had ever been awarded on a test and high points of the day for their division.

In his remarks, the judge had, "Nothing to add."

Timor eventually went back to his home, and then life became busy for his owner. As can happen, the duties of motherhood and her career took its toll on her time with her horse. He was alone in his paddock much of the time, which was too much for the Morgan. Timor finally took matters into his own hooves: He ran away and headed back to Heidi's farm, not once, but *five* times within a two-week period. His message came through loud and clear: Timor wanted to be reunited with his herd.

Heidi was concerned that all the rearing and chasing between Mike and Timor would start up again. She wondered if we could use Horse Speak to reintegrate the herd.

Hello?

I had informally helped multiple horses integrate with each other before, but it had never been the predominant reason for my work with a client, so this was interesting. I figured I should start by saying hello and see what

Greeting showed me about the black Morgan that wanted to be back with this herd.

I met Timor outside his stall, and we sailed through all three Greetings. When it came time for the next of the Four Gs (Going Somewhere—see p. 45), I began with the Go Away Face Button. Before I want to literally *go* somewhere with a horse, I need to make sure all the Buttons work, and I want to see how the horse responds to his own protocol. Going Somewhere needs to be *together*, and I have watched plenty of Mentors school a young or confused horse by going through the Buttons endlessly until the student finally understands this rule.

Let's just say Timor's Go Away Face Button was broken.

AHA MOMENT

Timor had no idea what I was talking about when I pointed at his Go Away Face Button. No wonder Mike spent six weeks rearing and chasing him! I got a short crop to use as an extension of my arm so I could reach over and touch his Go Away Face Button, because he thought maybe he should rear in play with me like he did when he was annoying Mike. I needed to be clear about standing at a 45-degree angle to his shoulder, and I needed to aim slowly and deliberately *until he twitched an ear*. I repeated this lesson by taking my hand and crop away, stepping back from the stall, and then stepping back up, doing a Check-In, and asking for Timor's Go Away Face Button to move over. Rinse, repeat. I did this about 15 times before he finally understood. Then he did an "Aw-Shucks" and licked and chewed. The Morgan retreated into his stall to think, and Heidi and I retreated to talk it over.

This encounter potentially cleared up half a dozen confusing things about working with this horse. He never pinned his ears or tried to strike, but he gave the impression that he was only following the lead rope because he hoped you had something neat you wanted to do with him. At any moment, if Timor had other ideas than yours, he was not at all afraid to share them. However, he was also the first horse to leave grass and run up to anyone who came to the gate, hoping to have some fun adventure.

After allowing him a few minutes rest, I initiated a Check-In, and this time, when it was time for Go Away Face, Timor offered it first. He also wiggled his ears and bobbed his head a little. The effect was like that little brother saying, "I got it…I got it! It's Go Away Face! I knew that all along, I was just seeing if you did."

We had kept the other horses from the herd in the barn, too, so they could watch and see I was trying to reach the Morgan. They all began licking and chewing and snorting—it was like the whole team was applauding. Mike looked at me with big eyes, perky ears, and wiggling lips. I felt like he was saying, "You see what I have had to deal with? Whew!"

Next Step

The next step was to move the whole herd out to a side paddock while Timor was in the riding ring adjacent to it. I wanted to work with the whole herd first, so Timor could watch me talk to the Buttons on all his buddies. I hoped this would sink in. The little gelding's owner was there with Heidi, watching the process.

Timor trotted back and forth along the fence line separating him from the herd, until I approached Mike. Then he stood stock-still and watched. I went to Mike first because he was the Leader and Mentor. I was not going to dominate Mike or diminish him in any way. He had to live with Timor, and I wanted to show them both that I was there to help that happen. Mike was a little sensitive to any sort of stick, so when I approached with the short crop, I used it to scratch his chest after allowing him to sniff it. Then Mike and I sailed through the Greeting and he performed a very dramatic Go Away Face (I felt it was aimed at his young student across the fence!). Then, I stepped back and moved off to Greet the other horses. They all did three fast, huffing breaths on the back of my hand, and I blew softly toward their muzzles, too. Everyone offered an easy Go Away Face, with one horse using it as an excuse to move quietly away. This was a quiet and respectful moment between us. I knew these horses pretty well by that point and recognized they normally interacted a little differently than they were today. I was sure this was for Timor's sake, as well. Horses model behavior for each other to learn from. The herd and I were coming together to try to help this little guy get a clue.

I used the crop as an extension of my arm to signal to everyone one at a time to move their front ends over. Standing a good 6 feet away from each horse, I pointed the crop at the Mid-Neck Button and then down to the Shoulder Button (see p. 42). This simply asks a horse to step aside. Some stepped aside one step; others left. Next I aimed the crop at the Girth Button of every horse. As each horse flinched, lifted or dropped his head, or made some other acknowledgement of my aim, I lowered the crop and made an "O," blowing out and using an "Aw-Shucks" and deep rib breathing to tell them both collectively and individually, "Thank you, that's lovely."

I wanted them to know I was asking the group to stick together and move with my suggestions, not run away from me. They had all made some acknowledgment back, so I swung the crop out behind the Hip-Drive Button and rhythmically swished it up from the ground to the height of the Button. Have you ever seen a horse "swish" his neck toward another herd mate to tell him to get going? This was the motion I was trying to emulate. I wanted to say, "Move off now…but easy does it."

The whole herd moved off to the left, so I "dropped it to stop it": all cues down, "O" posture, and I added a little sitting motion, bending my knees and lowering my hips. The herd stopped. We all breathed, licked and chewed, and did "Aw-Shucks," with the whole herd dropping their heads low. Timor was riveted. He had not moved an inch. I again moved the whole herd a little more left, then right, and then about 20 steps forward.

Timor stared the whole time. It was his turn.

The Lion's Den

Timor sauntered over to me and stood ready for…something. He sailed through a much softer Greeting, and offered stiffly to move his head a little sideways. I took it; good enough. Now, I applied the Mid-Neck and Shoulder Buttons from a few inches away, still using the crop. Timor made a tiny little hop with his front end, and I made a loud snap with my fingers and pointed firmly at the Go Away Face Button.

He had asked: "Can we play? I love to rear!"

I had said: "No way."

He did his best Go Away Face, still stiffly, but at least he knew what to do. Again, I asked his front end to move over a little. He struggled to comprehend how he should move it if he wasn't moving it up in the air in a play rear. He looked really "stuck," so I changed to the Back-Up Button instead. This triangle-shaped point where the horse's front leg meets the bulk of the shoulder is full of nerves. Timor quivered and moved one foot backward. I heard snorts, neck shaking, and licking and chewing from the herd in the paddock next door. It was as though they were cheering him on.

We repeated this new lesson with his front-end Buttons until just aiming my pointer finger in the air at them was enough to have the Morgan lean, move, or soften…I took any positive response that wasn't "rear." Timor's owner admitted that his endless "play drive" had caused him to chase her. She would duck behind trees in his paddock—a game he found delightful. She kept him away with a whip in her hand, and he never hurt her in any way, but he just needed to play so badly. She didn't care for the game, and tried to find other activities to distract him, but often participated in his form of "chase" because she felt guilty about not spending enough time with him.

I explained that what passed for a high "play drive" was due in part to deep-seated confusion. Animals and humans alike learn through play; that is why childhood is all about it. He was using play to try to learn, but he was not understanding the lessons. By going very slowly and using repetition, I was getting Timor to use his brain to stay engaged while his body learned the lesson. It would take about 300 Go Away Face encounters to really sink in. It had taken Mike six weeks to put the Morgan in his place last time. If I could drive the new neuropathways home by using rhythmic repetition, he would retain this lesson better. There was a sameness to my motions that created a rhythmic pattern like a dance. Variety was not our ally right now.

Finally, I had Timor follow me, targeting my knuckles as I held an imaginary lead rope. This simulated his lead line skills, but by doing the exercise with him loose he could show me what confused him without the added stress of being attached to each other. In Going Somewhere horse protocols, the first step is, "Do you know the Buttons? Can you move off if I ask?"

Watch horses closely, and you will see them use the Go Away Face, Mid-Neck, and Shoulder Buttons, as well as the Back-Up Button for average, everyday conversations. It may seem like a question (if the horse asking is using enough "O"), or it may be a demand (if the horse is using enough "X"). Horses calibrate the level of intensity between their "asking," "telling," and "insisting" by increasing the potency of their "X" until they reach a Level Four (see p. 103 to review intensity levels). Level Four intensity requires a lot of energy, and nature tells horses to conserve their energy (in case they need to run), so horses try to keep conversations as "low calorie" as they can. Much of what looks like horses "just standing around" is communication. It may be as subtle as "hard" or "soft" glances toward each other, but you will begin to notice that horses aim for these Buttons. They spend a lot of time negotiating personal space, one single movement at a time. Going Somewhere included the 15 minutes they spent readjusting themselves a little bit here and there, before they picked up and walked off to a new location.

Timor was clueless about "low-calorie conversations," so before I brought another horse in, I wanted him to at least be dimly aware of his Buttons and how he was expected to react when they were activated. The little Morgan was now following my target hand, stopping when I stopped, "matching steps" (more or less) when I asked for it, and coming to me with a lowered head when I beckoned. The last thing I needed to check was how he would be when he moved out. Could he still pay attention to me at a faster gait, or would he tune me out or freak out with excitement?

I stepped toward the middle of the riding ring, swishing my hand by my side to tell him not to follow. He complied, staring at me. If nothing else, Timor was having fun. Aiming the whip toward his Girth Button, I asked him to move off. At first, he started to walk toward me, so I rhythmically swung the whip toward his Go Away Face Button, then down to the Mid-Neck Button. He got it and veered off toward the left. No panic or trouble so far. I asked his Hip-Drive Button to move a little faster. I had previously "made friends" with his hindquarters, so the Morgan picked up a nice trot as though we did this all the time. He flicked his ear onto me, and I "sat down" a little and flexed my core. He looked at me, arching his neck in response.

Great! I wanted to know if he was really paying attention, and his adaptation to my own change in posture showed he was.

Then I stomped my feet and dropped all cues, making an "O." Timor stopped short and turned to face me, but stayed where he was. Although I knew he had worked on the longe line and at liberty before, it had been a few years, and knowing that he had taken to chasing his owner meant I really wanted to make sure I had his mind "with me" before introducing another horse to the scenario. I was getting ready to bring Mike in.

Before that, however, I had Heidi go over all the basic groundwork with first the herd and then with Timor. This was *her* herd, and I needed to transfer the balance of authority back to her. I also wanted to clear up any confusion she may have had.

She sailed through the basics, and the horses all licked and chewed and snorted, blinking eyes and wiggling lips and doing "Aw-Shucks" whenever she did. They moved around calmly and thoughtfully for Heidi, and Timor enjoyed practicing his newly discovered Go Away Face Button.

So far, so good. It was time to bring in Mike.

Little Brother Grows Up

Mike entered the pen, and we turned him loose, standing back to watch what he did when he reintroduced himself to Timor. They did a three-part Greeting, but it was very fast, and they repeated it three times, with a long linger on the last sniff—and then *bam*…right up into rearing. The highly charged greeting was typical between horses that are in a hierarchy dispute, or between rowdy young males. This was why I had been asking Timor to practice his Greeting more slowly and more deliberately. There was a split second where Mike aimed at the Go Away Face Button, but Timor pulled his head backward and avoided it. Aha! I could see that Timor had gotten so good at avoiding Mike's attempt to reach his Go Away Face Button that he was never learning this essential lesson!

I had my answer, so it was time to break it up. As I entered the riding ring with them, Mike paused to acknowledge me, but Timor got in his face and continued to try to play. He reminded me of one of those little dogs that yips and dances on its hind legs, wagging its tail furiously and licking people's legs, hands, faces, or whatever is closest. If Timor could have yipped and wagged his tail like that, he would have.

I made three changes of direction in front of them by walking a few steps, stomping my feet, and then turning around. I also kicked a traffic cone that happened to be in the ring. Mike came to a stop, and pinning his ears, bit Timor hard on the Mid-Neck Button. Timor yielded away, then finally seemed to notice me. I asked them both to come do a Greeting by holding both my hands at arms' length, knuckles up, toward them. Mike hesitated, glancing at Timor (it looked like a calculated glance) then marched over and Greeted me. Timor held back at first, but when I asked Mike for a Go Away Face, Timor came over—he recognized it as his new thing, too. The Morgan touched my knuckles, but his head was too high, so I backed up, made an "O," and blew out. Then I re-extended both my knuckles. Mike and Timor walked together to the Greeting, and Timor's head was lower now. Touches one, two, and three were a little too fast for my liking, but okay enough. I stepped sideways, aiming my shoulder toward Mike's shoulder to signal that we should "buddy up," and then I did a Shuddering Breath, blinking my eyes. Timor watched, as Mike did an "Aw-Shucks" in response, blinked, and snorted.

I had said to Mike: "Stick with me. I have a plan to cool things down."

Mike had said, "Great, I'll follow your lead."

Timor said nothing but tried to initiate play with Mike again. Swiftly, I stepped in. I had a short crop with a plastic bag tied to the end with me for this part. I swished it once toward Timor's Go Away Face Button, but I had angled myself between the two horses, so Mike would know that the bag swishing was not directed toward him. This is called "splitting the herd." Mike moved off a bit, tucking in behind me, while I stood my ground. Timor took a few surprised steps sideways, but was not all that affected by the bag. He was far too playful to be intimidated. As soon as he could, he reached out to try to snatch it in his teeth, and I had to use it to a Level Three ("telling") and then Level Four ("insisting") to make him yield his front end away—which he finally did (about 2 feet). As soon as it's over, it's over. I tucked the crop-and-bag down by my side, made an "O" posture, and told him he was a good boy.

Timor licked and chewed and eyed the bag down by my side with eagerness. All he was thinking was, "That looks cool and fun to play with. Can I try it?"

We all laughed.

I snapped my fingers toward the Morgan's Go Away Face Button instead of using the crop-and-bag, and he registered that better. I put the crop-and-bag outside the fence and got a small-sized longe whip with a tail. Since Timor had responded to the snapping of my fingers, maybe the sound of the whip tail would work better for him. This was *not* better for Mike, however. He immediately left the area as old fears of the whip surfaced. Timor went with him, and I had to start all over again.

Returning to the simple crop (without the plastic bag), I marched over to the two tussling horses and split them up by aiming first at Mike's Go Away Face Button and then at Timor's. I sent them both off at a trot by swinging the crop toward the Mid-Neck Button, all the way to the Girth Button.

Not only did I need to help Timor figure things out, I had to help Mike come up with better solutions, and I had to include Mike's leadership with my own to do that. Having them trot around together because I asked was better than watching them rear in front of me.

I moved in tandem with my shoulder aimed at Mike's. If I stayed in a small circle on the inside of the riding ring, I could adjust my timing and foot movements to "match steps" with him. By aiming my shoulder toward him, I was asking that we buddy up while we went. Mike caught on quickly, slowing his speed and cocking his ear toward me. I stepped out in front of his motion, blocking his front, and made a dramatic "X." Mike veered around the other way, and Timor followed Mike. Again, I "matched steps" at speed, slowed Mike down, and asked for a turn. We did this three times, and then Timor scooted past the last turn so that he was running away from Mike and me. Coming full circle into our path in only a moment (the little Morgan was very fast!) Timor watched to see what I would do. Ignoring Mike, I stepped firmly toward Timor and aimed at his Go Away Face Button with a firm snap of my fingers. The gelding veered around and took off, back in the same direction as Mike, who was still trotting along at a comfortable speed. This was all about Timor now, so I aimed at Mike's Yield-Over Button on his stifle, bent over into a quick "O," and stepped toward him in one, fluid motion. This told Mike to yield his hind end over and away, turning and facing me. He did this in a flash, and when I stepped three steps backward, beckoning to him, he moved toward me. I quickly swished my hand-tail at him and turned to trot off with Timor, who was still moving. Mike stopped in the center of the ring and stood there at Zero.

Now Mike and I were a team. If Timor wanted to join our team, he had to change his attitude. I knew he was super playful, and of course there could be some room for that, but he could not annoy the herd all day long.

I asked Timor to change directions several more times; to stop, start, come to me, move away from me, and so on. We had a Check-In near where Mike stood in the middle, and I would Greet Mike, too, but not allow Timor to play with him (which was just fine with Mike).

Finally, I had Timor standing near Mike. The draft cross was totally Zero: drooping his lips, blinking, and flopping his ears sideways. Timor looked at Mike, then at me, then released a long out-breath as he went into an "Aw-Shucks." I bent over and touched my toes, breathing out also. I wanted him to know he was totally welcome here, in a state of relaxation, and he would not be alone. He only ever felt connected with high voltage—I wanted him to feel connected in a "low-calorie moment," too.

For the first time, I moved in to scratch the Morgan's withers, chest, and belly. We were finally at the next G: Grooming. I think of Grooming protocols more like the social grooming you see in primates. It is not always about the physical touch, but instead the soft encounter of another body at peace. Timor leaned into my touch and almost forgot himself, nudging me for a moment. I held up my pointer finger toward the Go Away Face Button, and he snorted and straightened out his head.

Standing near him, but not touching, I began to "Rock the Baby" lightly by swaying from side to side. Soon, the horse adjusted his feet, nodded his head, and took a nap.

Hooray!

Big Mama in the Herd

We were now ready to turn everyone loose together in the larger pasture. One by one the horses in the herd were released in the field until it was Timor's turn. I had Heidi ready with a crop-and-bag (even though it didn't work especially well with Timor, it moved the other horses away just fine, and she decided it was the best tool for her to stay Zero).

The Morgan raced around the field at top speed, seeming to enjoy himself. The other horses ignored him. Even Mike did not race off to stop or redirect him. Another horse with Leader-type qualities made a face toward Timor when he scooted by, but it was one of the more timid horses in the herd—the usual low man in the pecking order—that pinned his ears and commanded Timor stay on the outside of the group if he was going to be silly. Herds are interesting, nuanced collectives. When you watch them, you learn something new every day.

Heidi needed to be the Mother of the herd for the last stage to happen. The boys were doing their best to ignore or tell Timor what to do, but without a Mother, there was no one for Timor to truly connect with. We all laughed and joked about Heidi being "Big Bag Mama"—her husband would be so pleased later to learn of her new title.

Heidi walked into the field with her crop-and-bag, and approaching the herd, swished lightly at the horses' Buttons. They all moved off according to which Button she signaled. Some turned to face her. She then did a Shuddering Breath, sighed loudly, blinked her eyes, and wiggled her lips. One by one (minus Timor who was still racing around on his own), the horses in the herd snorted, swaying their tails rhythmically, which meant they felt peaceful.

Finally, Timor came to see Heidi. He was careful to scoot around the main herd and approached her with a lowered head. She greeted him, then pointed at some grass and licked and chewed. The crop-and-bag was behind her back. Feeling more and more comfortable as I coached her, she didn't need the plastic bag anymore. Timor looked where she pointed and started eating near her feet. She tossed the bag aside and began to "hunt grass" with him. This is a ritual of connection between mothers and foals: the moms look for the best bites, and the foals eat what she is eating. By looking, pointing, and remaining in "O" posture, Heidi was filling the Morgan's need to be connected while eating. This was one reason he raced around and refused to settle down. He was not allowed to join the group, but without an eating partner, he couldn't relax. It was a catch-22.

After about five minutes with Timor, Heidi swished her hand-tail and marched off to join the herd. She spent a few minutes with each horse, hunting grass and being interested in what the horses were interested in. When we can make hunting grass an ally in our relationship and not an enemy (how many of us were taught to never let them eat grass when they are with us?), then finding food is a fantastic conversation you can share.

Soon, Timor had ventured nearer to the group. The same timid horse that had told him to stay away earlier still wouldn't let the Morgan come closer, so Big Mama (Heidi) stood up tall, pointed at that horse, and snapped her fingers, telling him to step back. When he did, a ripple went through the whole herd. It was as though a warm vibration affected everyone; even the onlookers. A deeper level of Zero was hitting us all. Our nervous systems are much more complicated and interesting than we often consider. When you are surrounded by horses and they all drop into Zero like that, it is unmistakable.

Heidi did not encourage Timor to get any closer, but her presence in the group was firm. Big Mama said, "Let Timor graze near you, and leave him be."

And that was that.

Heidi left the field, and all the horses sorted themselves out now that she was not there, but it was quiet and uneventful. Every so often, Timor would leave the group to walk past us—he was looking to see where Big Mama was. Satisfied when he had her located, he would go back to grazing.

Timor's owner was thrilled to see that the little Morgan had finally grown up—even a little bit. And in the following days and weeks, the herd remained calm. There were momentary play sessions, but Timor could follow the lead of the others in the group. He felt connected now. He didn't need to have everything "high voltage" to know he was included.

LICK AND CHEW

Horse Speak body language helped Riley with his self-carriage so that his underlying "habit" could be exposed for what it was. Once that habit was addressed with body language that he could understand, he was able to address his carrying capacity himself. It only took the occasional body language reminder to encourage him to use himself better.

When it came to Timor, the pivotal moment was when I realized the little Morgan had *no idea* what the Go Away Face Button even meant. I can only speculate as to why he didn't understand it; but the bottom line was that without understanding this core concept of horse protocol, he could not settle down into the herd or inside himself. Timor desperately needed to find his Zero again, but with a whole Button missing, how could he?

Horse Speak helped fill in the blanks.

Chapter 14

The Mare Who Said "NO"

I was invited to work with a local breeding stable and help their staff and trainers find Zero with their horses. There were quite a number of beautiful animals at this establishment: several stallions and a bevy of mares and foals. The stable often sold green horses just started under saddle, and frequently the horses went on to careers in the show ring.

While all the people who worked at this establishment had a deep love for the horses, there can tend to be quite a lot of energy in such places, and horses of pedigree can easily get worked up.

I was to spend part of my day at the farm with two mares that needed attention. One mare would often freeze up, and although she would stand perfectly still, her skin would shiver at the slightest touch. The other mare seemed to be in a state of perpetual stress, vacillating between needy and seeking attention and aggressively demanding her own way. There were also several other horses in their stalls at that time, and I was to meet and give a quick assessment about each one.

As you've seen in other stories in this book, the Greeting ritual can be used to diagnose quite a lot about a horse or to at least give you a heads up about his state of body and mind. Many of the horses had fairly consistent Greetings: neither excessively pushy nor overly nervous. I worked with one mare in particular that gazed back at me after completing Go Away Face with a look of tremendous interest. She eagerly did a Check-In with me, then sniffed toward my neck and performed a full, quiet circle in her stall, finishing with another Check-In. She was basically telling me, "I like you! Here are *all* my Buttons. Let's get together and talk!"

Her name was Celeste.

Chatty Mama

Celeste was a beautiful mare and the proud mother of several babies. She came out of her stall with a regal and lovely attitude, stepping exactly in time with every single step I made ("Matching Steps"). If I stopped and backed up, she caught her hoof in mid-air to amend its landing site so it fit exactly with mine. This was a horse that had schooled many children and was an excellent teacher, which was why she was so happy to follow my ideas. After walking up and down the aisle for a few minutes, lost to each other's dance, we finally landed ourselves at the end where the session participants were waiting.

There was an area near the wash stall that was wide enough to allow moving a horse comfortably around, so I focused the clinic there. It was quite cold outside, and this was a nice alternative to being in the wind.

One by one, Celeste performed the Greeting ritual with each person there, while I held the lead rope and acted like a guide. She paused and waited for the participants to remember what came next and when—even prompting those who forgot. It became very clear that Celeste had taken over and was the master of her own language. She wanted to repeat the Greeting ritual a second and even *third* time, offering to linger with anyone who was interested.

When it was time to "Match Steps" with her, practice lead rope skills, and learn to use awareness to create proper balance in turns and stops, Celeste made learning fun and easy. The barn manager laughed and commented that it must have been difficult for the mare to put up with how bumbling all the human beings were!

All in all, Celeste was not only chatty, but truly a horse at Zero. She embodied all the best natural grace and charm that a horse at peace within herself had to offer. Her life had been full, happy, and proud, and she was now eager to escort her human friends into a new chapter.

Faraway Mary

After lunch, we returned to the barn. It was time to work with the two troubled mares. For all that Celeste had to offer, these two mares were on the opposite end of the stick.

Both horses been acquired from other stables, and although they had each had a few babies and were deemed excellent mothers, they had a hard time with human beings.

I worked with the fearful, "frozen" mare first, hoping her story was a little simpler to sort out. Oftentimes, if you repeat the Greeting ritual often enough, and then use it to Greet all the objects and elements in the horse's world—such as the halter, brushes, doorways, thresholds, and so on—frozen horses warm up in the trust this creates.

The mare's name was Mary, and she held herself stock-still in the back of her stall as I approached. I blew a soft, huffing breath toward her three times to invite connection, and she finally acknowledged me with a slight look. She then took one, deep breath in and carefully approached the stall window. This was a good sign. It meant that she was not so lost inside herself that she didn't even want to try.

We completed all three nose-to-knuckle touches, and she offered a long, slow, Go Away Face, then blew out her nose and sauntered back to the other side of her stall. She had said hello, and now she was done.

I couldn't argue with that. It was polite, sincere, and very clear. You cannot force relationship, so I simply moved on to the other mare for the time being.

The second mare, named Hera, came careening to the window too quickly and with mixed messages. At first, her ears were perky and interested, and just as fast, they were laid back and her expression turned sour. It was as though she was saying, "Yes!" and "No!" at the same time. I have witnessed many Mentor horses deal with this sort of intensity, and it is always with a very quiet answer. So I remained out of reach unless I bent forward to extend my knuckles to Greet her. Even though she rolled her eyes and pinned her ears, she reached forward, too, and touched my knuckles. Everything in this mare said she was both desiring connection and fearing it. I didn't know her history and usually ask people not to tell me so I am not distracted by outside thoughts when I meet a horse. I wanted Hera to tell me about herself.

I stepped back to give her space. As you've learned in earlier chapters, horses value personal space above all other things, so by giving her breathing room, I was proving to her that I understood and respected this. I looked to the side and examined the stall next door for a few moments. By checking out the environment, I showed her that I was concerned about the same kinds of things she might be concerned about. I was trying to create a bond. Nodding my head to signal my intention to approach again, I blew out a relaxing breath and stepped up to the stall window for the second touch. She had been watching me the whole time, and now she also moved forward to reach my knuckles. She was still very defensive, but also curious, and offered the slightest inhale of the scent of my hand.

Stepping back once again, I walked off, not wanting to push the third touch yet. I wanted to impress upon Hera that I was not going to demand anything of her. After a few minutes, I walked back to her window and extended my knuckles. She tentatively reached over, almost despite herself, and touched the back of my hand, then rapidly pulled her head back and pinned her ears, retreating to the back of her stall.

I was encouraged by this small gain. Many horses in Hera's state of stress and confusion would not offer the third touch; at least she was trying. I sauntered off to revisit Mary.

Surfacing

Mary had watched my interaction with Hera and now was waiting at her window for a Check-In with me. She reached down and sniffed my knuckles, lightly lipping them. Removing my hand, I asked her for a Go Away Face and stepped away myself. This may seem counterintuitive, but proving to her that I was more concerned with space than touch would go further than reaching out to try and pet her.

Mary took my cue and lifted her head high, staring at the back door. I followed her gaze and stared hard at it, including a Sentry Breath and licking and chewing to say I thought all was clear. She continued to stare, so I joined her in staring, as well. Only a moment later, the door opened, and in walked on of the barn hands. She stared fixedly at him, then darted back into her stall. Pointing toward him as he went about his business, I said out loud, "Don't come any closer."

The poor guy looked up and asked what I was talking about. I told him this horse was anxious, and I was just trying to convince her I would help her feel safer. He laughed nervously and admitted that he was anxious around her, too.

Mary had watched me the whole time, and now stuck her head out of the stall to look at the man again. I asked him to look down for a second and breath out. He was a "good egg" and did so. Instantly, Mary did, too.

There were several participants near me so I asked them all to look down and breath out. They all obliged, and Mary quickly looked to them and did the same. The message was universal: Let's all take a big breath and start over.

I thought Mary could be one of those horses that was so sensitive that any ripple of emotion sent her into a panic. It would help her if she could feel more connected to people; she would tolerate human feelings better if she was not interpreting everything humans did as bad.

Asking the group to step forward, I encouraged everyone to Greet Mary with three quick touches. In this case, I had already done the more formal Greeting, so a faster "Hello," would work well for everyone else. At first, the mare was unsure, but by the third person, she got into the swing of it, and even reached out for people after that. Her eyes brightened up, and her nostrils began to flare as she took in people's scents.

I asked the group to go through the line one more time and this time do a simple Check-In with a Go Away Face to assure her they all intended to follow the rules. Not only did she eagerly Greet everyone the second time around, she moved her face elegantly away with only a slight suggestion she should. The second-to-last person forgot to ask her to move her face, and Mary stared at her, breathing and waiting. Someone else reminded the woman to ask for Go Away Face, but the woman had a kind disposition and admitted she didn't want to ask the mare to take her face away. As she half-heartedly lifted her finger in the air like the other people had, Mary refused to move. I told her that Mary didn't believe her, and was waiting for her to actually mean what she said. I told the group that "gray areas" were this horse's worst nightmare and that inconsistency would scare her.

The woman tried again, but before she could even lift her finger, Mary had elegantly turned her head aside, while keeping her eye on the woman. I asked the woman to check in with her feelings and determine whether or not she sensed that Mary was offended in any way. She replied that far from feeling offended, she actually felt quite connected to Mary, and could see that Mary was still watching her. At that, Mary swung her face back around, and gently sniffed the woman on the shoulder with a surprising amount of tenderness. In response, the woman reached up to pat Mary, and the horse shot backward as though she had been shocked.

I explained to the group that unwelcome touch is harder for horses to deal with than the Go Away Face Button, which clears up the confusion of respect for personal space. If we want to link petting with emotional plea-sure for a horse, it has to come *after* the conversation about space has been sorted out.

The last person in the group performed a very clear Greeting and Go Away Face, including stepping backward and looking down the aisle to tell the "bogeyman" to stay away. Mary turned to look at the door as the participant was pointing at it, then blew out her nose and put her head down low, licking and chewing. The person then stepped up and offered to pet Mary on her fore-head, which can be a friendly spot (see p. 42). Mary tolerated it for a moment, then turned her head away—but slowly.

This was a very good sign. I asked everyone to step back and opened the stall door three times in a row. Each time I stepped into the opening, then out, before shutting the door. The first two times, Mary shivered and jumped with every little sound. The third time, she blew out her nose, and dropped her head down in an "Aw-Shucks."

I grabbed her halter and lead rope, and stepped inside to Greet her nose with them three times in a row. Once again, on the third time, she put her head down in an "Aw-Shucks," and even shook her neck a little, releasing some stress.

I closed the door and turned to the group, explaining that I was using the Greeting ritual with both the door and the halter. Approaching and retreating from Mary three times in a row made my actions predictable, so whatever this horse had experienced in the past that caused her to be so overreactive would be less of an obstacle to creating a new connection with me. Mary was not seeing *me* as I was; she was reacting to her expectations of human beings, based on previous experience.

Thawing the Ice

I do not assume that a horse has been abused simply because he is overreac-tive. Certainly, abuse will cause this, but some horses are so sensitive and have such strong instincts that they simply cannot tolerate human inconsistency. What may be mildly annoying to a more stoic horse is wildly unsafe for a very sensitive soul.

Human beings are inconsistent en masse. We may one day feel that having a horse rub his head on us is fine and even welcomed, and the next day, we will feel the horse is rude or even angry about it. Horses have a way to ask each other what is welcome and what is not, and are very clear about what they do and do not want. The primary need for personal space trumps all other needs. In the case of two horses that are close in the pecking order, you can often see minor disputes all day long, but even those tend to be display and not so much contact. When horses *are* making a good deal of contact, it often points to one of two things: either their play drive is excessively high and they cannot get off the subject (think of Timor in the last chapter), or their insecurity is excessively high, and they tend to drive others in the herd crazy as they constantly seek comfort and safety.

With Mary, the barn staff assured me that she was higher in the pecking order among the other broodmares; it was only with people that she shuddered and "froze." My concern in working with Mary was that frozen horses can react in surprising ways when they unfreeze. I have been on the receiving end of such a wake up, and I prefer to avoid that if I can. However, I can usually tell when a horse is calm and steady versus when he is in internal panic. Generally, a truly frozen horse (as opposed to just "still") has a faraway look, a tense mouth, and reacts with a lot of skin twitching and flinching at the slightest noise or touch, though they do not make a move. These horses are frequently mistaken for being good school horses or are bought by unsuspecting new owners because they seem so calm on the outside. A frozen horse may wake up at any time, though, depending upon his reasons for freezing in the first place.

I returned to the stall to see how my initial Greetings were working out for Mary. The mare met me at the window, and delicately touched my knuckles three times. Her eyes seemed larger, softer, and made direct contact with mine. I blinked at her, and she blinked back at me, adding a Go Away Face. Blinking took the pressure off; her ability to blink back at me meant she was understanding me.

Opening the stall door, I placed the halter on her head, and she held still for it but maintained eye contact. Eye contact is actually important with horses. They look each other in the eye all the time and use "eye messages" in much the same way we do. How often is there a silent scene in a movie in which the actors convey all that is needed with only their eyes? Horses are like this, too—we have to use soft eyes and blinking to stay connected. Hard eyes leveled on a horse drives him away.

Once Mary was on the lead rope, I asked her other front-end Buttons to do three different things: First, I used my palm to ask her Buttons to *stay with* me or even *lean into* me. Second, I used my pointer finger to ask those Buttons to *yield away* from me with a lean or even a step. Third, I used what I describe as a "coochy-coo" finger, which is the motion we use when signaling someone to follow by curling our finger up and making a drawing motion toward ourselves. In explaining this motion, I often suggest you envision pulling an imaginary string from the Button to yourself. In some cases, "coochy-coo" is enough to encourage a horse to at least lean toward you; in other cases, you may need to back up three or so steps to make space for the horse to step into. It is important when doing this drawing-in motion that you are in an "O" posture, which also looks beckoning.

Basically, I asked Mary, "Can you hold still, move away, and move toward me with your face, neck, shoulder and front feet?"

Then I asked her to do a single step of the Therapy Back-Up to release tension in her lower back and pelvis (see p. 115). She rounded her back nicely and stepped back lightly, but her ears pinned, and she made a tense face.

There are a few reasons why a horse may have this sort of reaction to the Therapy Back-Up. First, if he has been backed up as a form of punishment, then he will associate it with that. Second, horses take in the world through the senses of their face, but they sort out their feelings through their hind end. The tail expresses the end result of what their eyes, ears, nose, and mouth have received. Stored emotional tension is frequently locked into their hind end, so rounding the lower back and releasing it can send some surprising feelings rushing through them. I have seen this so often that I anticipate it, and with Mary, I was pretty sure there were going to be some stored feelings there. On a practical level, backing up was the opposite of running away, so by cutting off her escape route, I was also challenging her to trust me a little more. She didn't have a real reason to do so, and again, I didn't take this personally; rather I was searching for all the ways she lost her Zero. Backing up was one of them.

I was very quiet and calm, and asked for Therapy Back-Up a few more times, including a "hot potato" release with much deep breathing, licking and chewing, and stepping away from Mary when it was complete to give her room to think. My goal was to help her release a good deal of stress.

When I teach this exercise to others, I explain that the most important feature is letting go of the lead rope, stepping away, and taking a breath as soon as the *smallest try* has opened up. Getting people to *stop asking* is the hardest part of this kind of work, which is why staying Zero and learning to pause, breathe, and give some space back to the horse is so important.

The way horsemanship has been presented to the human race for at least the last hundred years is that it is fine to expect and demand obedience from a horse, and that by poking, prodding, clucking, swishing, and whipping, we will get a submissive animal that performs as we want. In many cases this can be true. We can beat horses into submission, and many will simply become the machine we are looking for. However, if we want to connect and have mutual respect and a real relationship with a horse, then we have to become much, much softer, slower, and more thoughtful. Horses are not beasts of burden in most of Europe and North America anymore. We do not ride into battle on their backs, ask them to plow our fields, or hunt our food with the help of their speed. Yet the tactics that would make a horse submissive enough to handle those situations are still commonly used. Modern horsemanship, for the most part, is about pleasure: The pleasure of winning a blue ribbon or of having an equine friend. If your friend came over to help you paint your living room, and when she arrived, you stuck a brush in her hand, pointed at the wall, and dropped the can of paint at her feet, she might turn around and leave. The better result is likely to be had if you paint alongside her, listen to music or chat, offer a beer and pizza for her effort, and thank her often.

If you want a horse to like you, then act likeable.

What makes this hard is that horses are huge. Our nervous system goes into high alert when a horse slips into hypervigilance and feels threatened. Our bodies tell us we could die if this animal freaks out. This is why offering Zero to the horse at every single juncture sends the message that it is the foundation—the platform from which all other things you do together spring. I want my horse to seek to stay at Zero because it is what I have modeled for him. And I want him to help me stay at Zero, too, sometimes! At the college where I teach and in therapeutic riding situations, I actively need horses to offer Zero to my students to help them learn. If the horse's nerves are tense and frayed, and the only way he can get through his day is by shutting down, then there is no mutual respect, and ultimately this is dangerous. This is how horses get sick, act out, and are more likely to hurt us.

Follow the Herd

After asking Mary to back up and come forward a few more times, she began to yawn. This was the ultimate sign of release, and it meant I was helping her let it go. By the time I opened the stall door wide for us to leave her stall, her ears were sideways, her eyes were soft, and her nostrils were breathing me in.

I stepped out of the stall with one solid footfall. Mary thought she could rush forward, as I was sure she was used to doing. Horses consider every single doorway, gate, and corner as a potential threat, because in nature, this is where predators lurk: behind thresholds. So I stepped back in again, then out, and back in again in big, loud steps. The mare's foot copied me perfectly, and a "light bulb" seemed to go off. She blew out her nose and shook her entire body.

Shaking off the freeze! I was very pleased!

Now, we could walk in tandem together, "Matching Steps" up the aisle. When it was time to turn around and walk back down the aisle, I pointed at her Mid-Neck Button and then curled my finger, asking her to draw that Button to me as I walked three steps backward, making space for her to turn in a well-balanced arc around my body, finding her own center of balance. Walking horses while holding their lead ropes too tightly or too loosely (with the horse following behind) sets them up to be unbalanced in their turns, and this is upsetting to them. Some people prefer horses to follow a few steps behind, and others prefer to have their horses' heads at their shoulders. This is neither right nor wrong ultimately. However, the manner in which you move your hand, arm, and body while with the horse affects where he uses his pivot point and what part of his body begins arcing first. If your hand is too low, the horse's upper neck bends first, and this unbalances his feet. If you hold him too high and tight, he will bend from his back, which is not possible, and so he will bump into you. If you are too unaware while leading out in front of your horse, then it is like hauling a trailer behind your truck that falls off the hitch and fish-tails all over the place.

Ultimately, using the Mid-Neck Button by touching it with your leading hand before you make a turn changes your own body position and orients your own bend, allowing the horse to understand how he should pivot. I also like to look into a horse's eyes when I'm leading him because I am constantly check-ing in to make sure he is present with me and not becoming fixated on some "bogeyman." I do not walk off as though the horse is a trolley I am dragging around nor do I haul the horse by his face. Placing my palm downward on the lead rope, I turn my core toward the Mid-Neck Button or his chest, then turn forward, telling the horse I want his core to follow mine. Using my feet, I ask him to follow my footfalls. If I must, putting the "scoop" into the lead rope helps create a light bend in the horse's body, which usually removes tension and allows him to feel safe following me (see p. 80 for about the "scoop").

I was a dog obedience trainer for several years. I competed in obedience matches and won blue ribbons with a hybrid wolf. This animal taught me how to bridge the gap between obedience and devotion. He was trained to obey hand and whistle signals, to jump hurdles, carry a backpack, and pull a sled. Yet none of that would have been possible without deep mutual respect. (And he lived with me in my house, so there were plenty of couch potato days, too.)

Dogs move in a pack with personal power—all pack members need to be sharp and ready to hunt. Horse herds move with personal power, too, but very differently. All members need to know where they are in relation to the other members, so they are ready to defend each other and themselves from hunters.

When I move a horse on a lead rope, I have cut off the horse's ability to escape. I cannot mask his fear of being hunted with obedience. I must address his need to stay balanced and engender a *sense* of freedom within him if I want him to choose to follow me. I have had many years working with troubled horses, and I can certainly wrestle with one if I have to…but I would much rather engage a horse's urge to follow the herd and set myself up as a good Leader to be followed.

I brought Mary back to her stall, and she blew her nose, lifted her tail, and released gas while shaking her whole body again. She then turned to the back of her stall and rested. Becoming embodied—experiencing the body in a feeling, conscious way—after a lifetime of being shut down can be exhausting.

Hera Says "NO"

Returning to Hera's stall, I attempted to do the same routine I used with Mary, opening Hera's door and greeting her with her halter three times. She responded reasonably well and allowed me to place the halter on her without too much fuss. Her usual handler was there, a young woman named Terry who was trying to learn Horse Speak, and she said that it was the easiest she had ever seen Hera be about haltering. But in my mind, Hera was a stewpot of stress. She would not blink with me, nor would she breathe or relax her poll. Sometimes I use a "Yes" or "No" nod of my head to ask horses to release the tension in the poll.

Hera said, "No."

I stepped back out of the stall and did an "Aw-Shucks" in the aisle. Hera stepped back and lowered her head, only to pop back up and charge the stall window with her teeth bared.

Hera had witnessed her friend Mary come out of her frozen state, but that was not cutting it for her. I wondered if she was more defensive in her stall due to the confinement. Terry said the mare was often much better outside. I decided to try a change of scenery.

Terry approached Hera using the Greeting ritual and staying out of her space much more than she usually would. Hera was quite edgy, but she knew Terry and trusted her. It is sometimes the case that a horse is so sensitive to "trainers" that as soon as he thinks I am one, he throws up all his defenses, and it is better in the long run to coach his regular handler instead of trying to find the breakthrough myself. This was already the case with Hera. I instructed Terry to offer her one long stroke from her poll all the way down her near front leg, then to step to the side a little. As soon as Terry offered this downward stroke, Hera blinked her eyes and pursed her lips in pleasure. Everything about this mare was so tightly wound, yet she was craving release. In most cases, touching a horse in distress is the worst thing you can do, as it adds to it. However, because Hera responded well to Terry's presence, I was hoping to deepen what was already working between them.

Terry did a fine job following my coaching and leading Hera using "Matching Steps" over the threshold of the stall and down the aisle. She was already good with her own body, so adding new awareness to leading Hera came naturally. When she touched Hera's Mid-Neck Button and asked the mare to pivot around her, Hera paused and seemed to get stuck. Terry told me the mare would freeze up like this sometimes. I encouraged her to use the "scoop-up" motion on the lead rope and keep stepping backward, inviting Hera to come toward her. The mare nodded her head, blew out a breath, and took a delicate and careful step toward Terry, followed by more tentative but well-thought-out movements. Hera was literally rounding a corner as she found her balance point.

When horses balance physically, they feel mental and emotional balance, as well. Hera was not very mentally or emotionally balanced, and this showed up in her erratic movements. Terry confessed that she often called Hera the "tap dancer," because her feet seemed to go everywhere all at once.

Mary's handler Melanie was leading her out of her stall, and both horses and handlers were doing well together. Lifelong habits are hard to break, but the handlers liked the feeling of connection they were developing, and the horses were making a supreme effort to keep their heads lowered and calm. No one was truly at Zero, but all were making good strides toward it.

We let the mares free in a paddock together to observe them. Mary went about checking the fence, sniffing for strands of leftover hay, and "scanning the horizon." Hera called for other horses, kept her head high, and trotted around nervously wringing her neck and tail. Finally, Hera settled in and came to Greet Mary, who had kept her head low the whole time. They did two touches, then Mary broke away to make a slow circle before coming back to greet Hera for the third touch. Hera immediately did a Go Away Face, and then pinned her ears and nipped toward Mary's Play Button on the side of her mouth (see p. 42). Mary pinned her ears in response and aimed "hard" eyes into Hera's Go Away Face Button along with a very sour grimace—but otherwise she did not move an inch.

Hera got the message and moved in a large circle, coming back to stand a foot or so away from Mary to do an "Aw-Shucks." Mary did a Go Away Face, leaned away, and started to move her feet slowly, too. Hera fell into line, slightly behind Mary. Hera wanted to push Mary to move forward faster—so Mary halted instead, lifting her head high and tightening her tail (making the horse version of "X"), telling Hera she would get a reprimand for trying to drive her. Hera ducked her head low again and turned to the side. She moved a few feet away, then targeted Mary's Girth Button with her eyes. Mary slowly moved off again, with Hera aimed to follow from her flank—this time, *not* in the drive position.

Mary moved to draw Hera's attention to several interesting spots on the fence line. She lingered on one spot long enough to get Hera to sniff the same area, then ducked her head down, shaking her neck and licking and chewing before walking off to another spot. After a few minutes of checking the fence, Hera had calmed down and headed toward the center of the paddock to roll.

I narrated the whole encounter to the clinic participants, explaining that Mary was using her lowest level "X" and scanning the environment to help Hera to be in the here and now and relax. Mary used slow movements, heavy steps, and lots of deep breathing. Hera jumped up after rolling to scoot quickly around the paddock, kicking out her heels. Mary adopted her "X" but stayed motionless as Hera ran around. She was holding down the Zero position in their herd of two and telling Hera that she was on the lookout, so she would not be sucked into any sort of play right now. Hera came back to Mary, lowered her head, and touched noses, breathing deeply. She flopped her ears to the side, and then used heavy steps herself to saunter off to look for the old strands of hay that were gathered here and there. Mary moved to the rolling spot, had a nice roll, and then stood up—no kicking or running for her. Hera stood calmly, watching Mary, and blew her nose once Mary was back on her feet.

I asked the handlers to go get two flakes of hay and toss them about 10 feet apart in the paddock. I knew what to do next.

As soon as each mare had claimed a hay pile, the two handlers and I went inside. We were going to simply approach one of the mares until we could see a flinch, then back away. We were going to do what I call the "Reverse Round Pen," in which you move in a complete circle around the outside of the horse's "bubble of personal space" while the horse does not move at all (see p. 49). Horses can ask each other to move, but they can also tell each other to stay still. For different reasons, this activity would do wonders for each mare and her handler.

It took about 10 minutes to complete a circle around the mares. The handlers needed to watch for any movement from the horse at all and back away as soon as they saw it. Once or twice, they pushed too far, and the horses walked off, changing hay piles. By the end of the lesson, the girls came away with a new appreciation for how sensitive horses really were and how each part of the horse's body had different levels of comfort.

I asked the handlers to approach their horses and offer a Greeting. Both mares lifted their heads halfway and softly greeted their girls. Mary snatched a large mouthful of hay and offered it to her handler Melanie, who was a bit surprised. Mary never offered things like that. I told Melanie to share the hay with the mare, picking it apart with her fingers. Horses will share hay with each other, and mothers allow their foals to eat out of their mouths.

Hera moved her head away from her handler's presence. I told Terry that she was "conceding" the whole pile to her and that she should move away. You don't want to make a horse feel driven from his hay pile; he can get sour about it. Once I have a good relationship with horses eating hay, I will sometimes drive them from one hay pile to the next in a soft, gentle manner to establish respectful hay interactions, as well as convince them I will make sure they get their needs met. Sometimes when I am working with herd integration, moving from hay to hay is the best way to demonstrate to the horses the manner in which I want them to eat dinner. I know that deep down, horses do not crave tension, so by modeling relaxed eating scenarios, I can often influence the herd to adopt new rules of conduct.

However, building up trust around food can be a tricky thing; I do not want a horse that is deferring space to feel driven away. As soon as Terry moved back, Hera swung her head toward the hay and then did a wonderful thing: She ducked her nose down and under a huge pile of loose hay and tossed it toward Terry. I told Terry to go to the hay that was offered and sort through it, finally tossing some back to Hera. The mare blew out her nose and flopped her ears sideways, blinking constantly. Both handlers stepped away from the horses.

Caring for many horses in a big stable means constantly being on the go. Both Melanie and Terry realized they had unconsciously seen horses having these sorts of conversations all the time, but never paid attention to it. They were overcome with warm feelings toward the two mares that they had not felt before.

Both mares had rounded their shoulders forward, and relaxed their bellies and floating ribs. They looked shorter and fatter as they both released deep tension. Their handlers commented they felt calm and peaceful inside.

I knew we were done for the day. Aiming everyone toward Zero was the goal, and horses and humans alike now had some new ideas and feelings about each other…and life. However, when Melanie began to move Mary toward the gate first, Hera began to get very upset very fast. She did not want to be left behind—she was looking for Mary to watch her back. This meant that Hera was still not giving Terry, her handler, the benefit of her trust…not quite yet. I stopped Melanie and Mary and asked them to walk around, sniffing fence posts instead, with Hera and Terry following. In about 10 minutes, Hera had calmed down, and we moved her to the gate first. Outside the paddock, she again became agitated and tried to dive for grass. Terry said this was all very unusual for Hera, who usually just walked around, sort of glazed over. I said we had woken the mare up and that, like Mary, she had been shut down internally, for whatever reason. Now Hera was awake, and she needed to talk about many things.

Terry had a hard time allowing Hera to snatch at the grass, fearing that the behavior would take over and become a bad habit. I told her that, in this case, the horse was in distress for reasons we couldn't understand, and we had to be at Zero, treating Hera the way Mary had treated her in the beginning of their time in the paddock. Snatching at the grass was a way for Hera to lower her head and try to get her composure back. I explained to Terry how to start taking over the mare's grazing, stepping heavily and solidly from clump to clump, and showing Hera where to go, just like they did when walking the fence line.

AHA MOMENT

The barn manager had been watching the work with the mares all day, and now she offered some additional insight. She informed me that Hera had been in the paddock we were using the day they sold one of her babies, and she had raced around and around for an hour, refusing to settle down. She said that Hera had reared several foals and never made a huge fuss when it was weaning time, but this baby was different. She seemed to be so attached to him, and a lot of her current stress had seemed to begin after that foal was sold. In fact, it had been so bad, they weren't sure they should breed her again.

No wonder Mary had taken such good care of Hera: She made space for the grieving mother to *just be*. Terry stepped solidly from one clump of grass to another, and Hera was now "Matching Steps" with her. The mare had changed from snatching angrily at grass shoots to nibbling gently, and she was blowing out her breath, even shaking her neck a little. I suggested that Terry aim for the mare's stall with her core and march her all the way there with surefooted assuredness to tell the mare she would have her back the whole way.

Day by Day

In the wild, mares form the bulk of the herd. There are grandmothers, aunts, mothers, and daughters, and they have very strong bonds. Young males are allowed to be in a herd if they do not try to breed or until they are old enough to go live with a bachelor band. Horses have very close family ties and separating them from each other can really knock them off their center. You can help a horse find his center again by finding Zero.

A few weeks later, I got a message from the barn manager. She was happy to report that both Hera and Mary were coming along. Mary had changed dramatically after the day I had worked with her and now was being used in riding lessons. This was a good outlet for her compassionate nature. Hera was being restarted under saddle, and they had decided not to breed her again. The two mares were turned out together every day, and the barn staff had begun to linger around their paddock to try and observe their interactions. For at least a few minutes every day, Terry now simply lingered with Hera, doing nothing but being still and present for her. Hera had developed quite an attachment to her handler and was starting to whinny when she saw her. The mare had a lot of old baggage about a great many things; however, the diligence and mutual respect was paying off, and day by day, she was letting go of stress and agreeing to more and more.

The rest of the staff who had been observing my Horse Speak clinic that day found themselves noticing tiny things that the horses did now, and overall the feel of the whole farm had found a kind of peacefulness. It was as though a ripple effect had gone through the place, starting with Mary and Hera and ultimately influencing all the horses.

Lick and Chew

Although commercial horse stables often have a business side that has deadlines and agendas, we can still find ways for the daily interactions staff has with horses to be soothing, nurturing, and supportive. Horses are okay with having a job to do and will just "do the thing" that we are asking of them. Like inviting that friend over to help paint the living room, if we are too task-oriented, we are losing out on the richness of life in that place where horses actually dwell. Horses in our modern world are filling a gap for us that has to do with feeling good…if we find a way to help them feel good as well, we all benefit.

Conclusion

Working with horses has been one of the most challenging and most rewarding things I have done with my life. It has been a great privilege and honor to be a part of others' journeys, and I am so grateful to the people and horses these stories are based on. There is no instant cure, fix, or type of training that takes the place of practice, sincerity, and authenticity. If nothing else, learning even a few "words" in Horse Speak may serve to bridge The Gap, wherever and whenever it shows up. Developing Horse Speak is a gift I hope to give back to the horses themselves, by making a sincere attempt to give horses a voice.

Thank you, my friends, my teachers, and my truest companions.

May the Horse Be With You!

Index

human healing through, 141–152.
See also human healing

with insecure horses, 169–182. *See also* insecure horses

keys to, 37–51. *See also* keys to Horse Speak

leadership, redefined, 9–10, 22–24, 44, 45–46

mindfulness during, 55–64. *See also* mindfulness

as new paradigm, 65–83. *See also* paradigm shift

nurturing, 213–230. *See also* nurturing conversations

partnership, redefined, 7–8, 29–31, 34

on releasing trauma, 121–139. *See also* post-traumatic stress disorder (PTSD)

on self-carriage, 193–201, 212. *See also* self-carriage

stages of, 45–46, 90

teaching vs. learning, 5–6, 8–9, 29

teaching vs. training, 167

horse whispering, demystified, 85–95

development of Horse Speak, 86–90

discovering Buttons, 85–86

teaching Horse Speak, 90–95

horsemanship philosophy, 13–35

anthropomorphism and, 14–16

on boundaries, 26–27. *See also* boundaries

catch phrases, 18

decoding and encoding, 20–22, 38–40, 94

"Hurry slowly," 25–26, 32–33, 39, 45

on making the wrong thing hard, 33–34, 69

on moving horse's feet for communication, 31–33, 49–51, 146–148

nature of language, 19–20

objectification vs. observation, 13–14

on postures, 24–25. *See also* "O" posture; "X" posture

on rapport, 16–17. *See also* rapport

on training, 27–31. *See also* training, redefined

Zero state for shared connection, 34–35. *See also* Zero, state of

human healing

background, 141–148

Zero state for, 148–152

"Hurry slowly," 25–26, 32–33, 39, 45

in-hand techniques, 61–62, 63

insecure horses, 169–182

background, 169–171

communicating with, 171–174, 181–182

leadership role with, 165, 176–182

"Interested Breath," 40

intimacy, 46, 49. *See also* mindfulness

Jag (horse), 88

Journey (horse), 153–164

Jump-Up Button, 131, 194, 196

keys to Horse Speak

breath messages, 40–41, 92, 100, 126, 128, 170–171, 176, 211

communication buttons, 41–45, 42f. *See also* Buttons

making the wrong thing hard,
33–34, 69
moving horse's feet for communication, 31–33, 49–51, 146–148
teaching vs. training, 167

wolves, 23

"X" posture
during conversations, 105–108,
119, 133–134, 157–160
description of, 24–25, 27
discovery of, 85, 87
with Hip-Drive Button, 44–45
horse version of, 44, 106, 225, 226
intensity levels for, 103–105,
157–160, 162, 164–166
while riding, 82

yawning, 77, 91–92, 102, 116–117, 137,
222
"Yes" message, 62–63

Zero, state of
with aggressive horses, 165–167
blinking and, 101
for boundary communication,
105–110
defined, 5, 11
healing and, 135, 148–152
intensity levels and, 103–105,
108–110, 165–166
paradigm shift and, 71–72
postures for, 24–25
with "Reverse Round Pen," 50–51
for shared connection, 34–35. See
also rapport
for stress release, 22, 24–26,
37–38
teaching vs. training, 167